RECOVERY
FROM SEXUAL ADDICTION:
A MAN'S WORKBOOK

RECOVERY
FROM SEXUAL ADDICTION:
A MAN'S WORKBOOK

Paul Becker, LPC

authorHOUSE®

AuthorHouse™
1663 Liberty Drive
Bloomington, IN 47403
www.authorhouse.com
Phone: 1-800-839-8640

Published by AuthorHouse   05/21/2012

ISBN: 978-1-4772-0212-8 (sc)
ISBN: 978-1-4772-0211-1 (e)

Library of Congress Control Number: 2012908267

Any people depicted in stock imagery provided by Thinkstock are models, and such images are being used for illustrative purposes only.
Certain stock imagery © Thinkstock.

This book is printed on acid-free paper.

Because of the dynamic nature of the Internet, any web addresses or links contained in this book may have changed since publication and may no longer be valid. The views expressed in this work are solely those of the author and do not necessarily reflect the views of the publisher, and the publisher hereby disclaims any responsibility for them.

Table of Contents

Acknowledgments viii

Introduction ix

Chapter One: My Sexual Behavior..1
  Men's Stories..1
  Andre's story 1
  Neil's story 1
  David's story 2
  Mike' story 2
  Ted's story 2
  Tony's story 2
  George's story 2
  James' story 2
 Pornography 4
 Masturbation...7
 Sexual Fantasy and Thinking 10
 Sexual Encounters 14
 Other Sexual Activities...17
 Legality/Job Jeopardy 20
  Your story 21
 Sexual Addiction Questions 25
 Am I Sexually Addicted? 28
 Your Summary 31

Chapter Two: Highlights of the Origin of Sexual Addiction 32
 Age-Inappropriate Exposure to Sexual Behavior or Material...................32
 Family Environment and Structure 32
 Arousal 33
 Feelings of Shame, Guilt, and Depression 34
 Learned Models in Childhood...35
 Your Summary 36

Chapter Three: Why Did I Become Sexually Addicted?..............................37
 Sexual Addiction Often Begins in Childhood...38
  Mark's story...38
  Your story...41
 For Some Sexual Addiction Has its Origin in Late Teen Years or Early Twenties 45
 Joshua's story—an alternative story 45
 Your story, an alternative story...46
 What Did I learn from the Last Two Chapters? 47
 Your Summary 48

Chapter Four: Why Can't I Just Stop? 49

   Altering the Brain and Forming a Habit...49

   Sexual Fantasies 52

   Your Acting-Out Environment 55

      Jude's story...55

      Your story 55

   Acting-Out Ritual...57

      Tom's acting-out ritual 57

      Your acting-out rituals 59

   Sex-Addiction Cycle 62

   Your Summary 67

   Are You Discouraged?...68

Chapter Five: Role of Anger, Anxiety, Depression and Isolation

   in Sexual Addiction 69

   Childhood Emotional Nourishment 70

      Ely's story..70

      Your family of origin..71

   Childhood Messages 73

   Role of Anger 77

   Role of Anxiety 80

   Roles of Depressed Mood 82

      Chronic depressed mood...82

      Your chronic depressed mood 83

   Addict's Life Scale...84

      Your life scale 85

      Next steps...86

   Role of Isolation 88

   Your Summary 91

      Keep in mind 92

Chapter Six: Codependency..93

   Codependency in Marriages Where the Male Is Sexually Addicted..............93

      Who is to blame? 94

   The Origin of Codependency Is Found in a Child's Dysfunctional Family..................95

   Children of Codependent Dysfunctional Families Have Ill-formed or

      Incomplete Personalities 95

   In Marriage, Codependency Fosters Pain and Negativity 95

   Codependency Addressed 95

      A visual picture of codependency relationship 96

      What needs to change?..96

Chapter Seven: Is There Hope? 100

  Salvation History...101

    King David...101

    Apostle Peter..103

    Apostle Paul...103

  Change the Dance...104

  Your Summary 105

Chapter Eight: Change the Dance..106

  Awareness and a Change of Attitude..106

  Summary Review 107

    Affect on my life...107

    The origin of my addiction 108

    Factors that keep me addicted...109

    Role of anger..111

    Role of anxiety...111

    Role of low-grade depression 112

    Role of isolation...112

    Exceptions..113

  Changing the Dance: New Steps...114

  Recognize That Addiction Causes More Pain than Pleasure 116

  Address Environmental Temptation..117

  Your Summary 118

Chapter Nine: Healthy Lifestyle..119

  Coming Out of Isolation..120

    Coming out of isolation by cultivating a strong male friendship..........120

    Coming out of isolation by improving family relationships................121

    Coming out of isolation by improving relationships with spouse and children 123

  Giving-up Depressed Mood 125

    Choose to take steps to live at a forty-point benchmark level 126

  A Close Relationship with God...128

    Change your relationship with God..129

  Develop a Support Network..130

  Your Summary 131

Appendix A: Interventions and Aids to Commitment......................132

    Which interventions did you choose?..136

Acknowledgments

To those who shared their stories—and only you know who you are—you will be indispensable to those who will benefit from sharing your journey.

I would like to thank and acknowledge Sherry Hart, Patricia Doane, and Dr. Ann Johnson who read drafts and made valuable and appreciated contributions to this endeavor.

God bless you all.

Other books by Paul Becker, LPC

Letters from Paul
In Search of Recovery: A Christian Man's Guide
In Search of Recovery Workbook: A Christian Man's Guide
In Search of Recovery: Clinical Guide
Why Is My Partner Sexually Addicted? Insight Women Need
Recovery from Sexual Addiction: A Man's Guide

The book, *Recovery from Sexual Addiction: A Man's Guide,* is a revised edition and replaces, *In Search of Recovery: A Christian Man's Guide. Recovery from Sexual Addiction: A Man's Guide,* adds substantial new material.

This book, *Recovery From Sexual Addiction: A Man's Workbook* is a revised edition and replaces, *In Search of Recovery Workbook: A Christian Man's Guide. Recovery From Sexual Addiction: A Man's Workbook* adds substantial new material.

To contact Paul Becker, e-mail: hh8326@gmail.com.

Introduction

This workbook is intended to help sexually-addicted men understand the origin of their addiction and to provide hope as they travel their recovery journey. It is intended to help men achieve the insight needed to make a high-level commitment to change their sexual behavior and thinking.

This workbook is a companion work to the book, *Recovery from Sexual Addiction: A Man's Guide*. While the book and workbook will facilitate individual counseling, they are best used as part of therapy with a competent therapist who has knowledge and understanding of sexual addiction. It will be particularly helpful to men in group counseling for sexual addiction.

This workbook contains a synthesis of material from multiple sources that I use in sexual-addiction counseling. When another author's material is used, credit is attributed.

Chapter One

My Sexual Behavior

If you are reading this book, you are probably struggling with the question, "Should I do something about my sexual behavior?" Let's review the stories of men who had the same question.

Men's Stories

Andre's story

Andre believed all men and some women enjoyed viewing pornography on the Internet. He felt nothing was really wrong with viewing pornography and engaging in masturbation. After all, he reasoned, "It really doesn't hurt anyone." Andre went on the Internet at his work site a couple times of a week, particularly after a long day. He looked forward to going on the Internet to view sexually stimulating images because he felt he deserved a little bit of enjoyment after having worked so hard. The IT department and his boss disagreed. He was fired.

Neil's story

Neil is married to Lisa. While Neil believes he and Lisa have an active sex life, he still feels drawn to self-stimulation. Several nights a week Neil tells Lisa he has work to do and stays up after Lisa has gone to bed. However, part of Neil's "work" involves going on the Internet to find sexually stimulating material as a precursor to masturbation. Neil believes his private life does not impact his marriage and his "arrangement" works. Neal is having a difficult time understanding why Lisa was so upset when she found him masturbating to sexually stimulating material late one evening. She insisted he seek help for his problem.

David's story

David is an ordained minister who was caught with a significant number of pornographic images on his laptop. While he feels relieved that his secret life was exposed, he expresses great fear that others in his congregation will find that he has feet of clay.

Mike' story

Mike looks forward to going to work each day. Mike rides the subway to work and he continually scans the car for young beautiful women on their way to work. At times he will engage a young woman in conversation in hopes it will lead to an encounter. Other times, particularly when the subway is crowded, he will stand close to a woman to facilitate body contact. His early morning ritual led to affairs and the last left him with a case of venereal disease.

Ted's story

Ted has a stressful job. Since his youth he has experienced high levels of anxiety. He is fearful he might not meet other people's performance expectations. Ted finds that masturbating a couple of times a day reduces his anxiety. Ted says he is not looking for sexual pleasure, just a reduction in his anxiety. He says he does it as fast as possible to get it over with.

Tony's story

In college Tony had a long distance relationship with Susan. They were only able to see each other a couple of times a year. However, they talked frequently on the phone and one of their pleasures was to talk dirty to each other. While the relationship did not survive the long distance, phone sex became a part of Tony's life.

George's story

George's first marriage ended in divorce. When George and Margie began dating, sexual activity was quickly introduced into the relationship. George said he now realizes he never became good friends with Margie; she was simply his sexual outlet. Today, George finds his life preoccupied with sex. He visits massage parlors, striptease bars, and he uses any form of sexual stimulation he can find. George told his therapist he feels lonely and wants to explore why.

James' story

As a child James lived in his head. He was an expert at video games and other forms of individual play. He said he frequently finds himself bored and turns to sexual fantasy to relieve his boredom. The most time consuming activity in which he engages each day is sexual fantasy and thinking. He wonders what it would be like to live a life free of sexual fantasy and thinking.

How about you? Do you identify with any of the men in these stories? Are you surprised to find you are not alone?

Perhaps your story is different. It is impossible to detail all the stories of men who wonder if they're dealing with a sexual addiction.

The following are questions which are intended to help you explore your story. These questions will help most men. However, if none of them relate to you, you will find a place at the end of the section to tell your story. What is your story? What behaviors are causing you concern?

Pornography

When did your attraction to pornography begin?

_____

_____

_____

When did your attraction to pornography become a concern to you?

_____

_____

_____

Do you view pornography on the Internet? Rent or purchase pornographic movies? View pay-for-view or TV porn channels? Read pornographic magazines? Exchange videos or images on the Internet? Use a cam camera to engage in or view sexual activity? Which one(s)?

_____

_____

_____

Are you aroused by images of straight sex, oral or anal sex, same sex partners, sadomasochism, younger/older women, or children? Which one(s)?

_____

_____

_____

What images of body parts are particularly appealing to you? This could be genitals—male/female, breasts, legs, hair, buttocks, necks, anorexic bodies, overweight bodies, etc. Which one(s)?

_____

_____

_____

Are you fearful of getting caught while viewing pornography?

_____

_____

_____

Do you view pornography in your home, workplace, Internet Cafe, other? Which one(s)? Why?

_____

_____

_____

Do you get aroused (mentally or physically) by images found on the Internet, commercial TV, magazines, newspapers, etc., which are not regarded as pornographic by the public in general? While the images may not be "pornographic," if the image causes you to be sexually stimulated, the image is pornographic to you. Which images(s)?

_____

_____

_____

How frequently do you view pornography? Why?

_____

_____

_____

What is the typical time lapse between viewing pornography? Why?

_____

_____

_____

Do you have a favorite time of the day during which you view pornography? Why?

_____

_____

_____

Do you find you are never satisfied with finding the latest pornographic image—you want more or better?

_____

_____

_____

Have you hurt someone in your life by viewing pornography? Who? How has it affected your relationship with that person(s)?

_____

_____

_____

Do you experience guilt or shame after you view pornography? Describe.

_____

_____

_____

Has pornography affected your spiritual connection to God?

_____

_____

_____

Have you tried to stop viewing pornography? Why?

_____

_____

_____

Have you been successful? If yes, why? If not, why not?

_____

_____

_____

Do you find you are able to stop for a while but sooner or later you find yourself going back?

_____

_____

_____

Do you want to end this behavior? Why?

_____

_____

_____

Masturbation

When did your attraction to masturbation begin?

_____

_____

_____

When did your attraction to masturbation become a concern to you?

_____

_____

_____

As an adult, do you masturbate?

_____

_____

_____

How frequently do you masturbate? Why?

_____

_____

_____

What is the typical time lapse between masturbation events? Why?

_____

_____

_____

Do you have a favorite time of the day during which you masturbate? Why?

_____

_____

_____

What stimulus do you use to masturbate? Do you use pornography, sexual fantasy, sex toys, or other aids to enhance arousal? Which one(s)?

_____

_____

_____

Do you find you are never satisfied after having engaged in masturbation and you seek more or better experiences?

_____

_____

_____

Have you hurt someone in your life by engaging in masturbation? Who? How has it affected your relationship with the person(s)?

_____

_____

_____

Do you experience guilt or shame after engaging in masturbation? Describe.

_____

_____

_____

Has masturbation affected your spiritual connection to God?

_____

_____

_____

Have you tried to stop masturbating? Why?

_____

_____

_____

Have you been successful? If yes, why? If not, why not?

_____

_____

_____

Do you find you are able to stop for a while but eventually you find yourself going back?

_____

_____

_____

Do you want to end this behavior? Why?

_____

_____

_____

Sexual Fantasy and Thinking

When did your attraction to sexual fantasy and thinking begin?

_____

_____

_____

When did your attraction to sexual fantasy and thinking become a concern to you?

_____

_____

_____

Is sexual fantasy and thinking an important part of your adult life? Why?

_____

_____

_____

Do you engage in sexual fantasy and thinking that consumes some part of your day?

_____

_____

_____

How frequently do you engage in sexual fantasy and thinking? Why?

_____

_____

_____

What is the typical time lapse between episodes of sexual fantasy and thinking? Why?

_____

_____

_____

What percent of the day do you engage in episodes of sexual fantasy and thinking?

_____

_____

_____

What body parts are particularly stimulating to you?

_____

_____

_____

In your sexual thinking or fantasy, is the subject of your fantasy a real person or just body parts to satisfy your lust?

_____

_____

_____

What do you use to stimulate your sexual fantasy and thinking?

_____

_____

_____

Do you have a preferred time of the day during which you engage in sexual fantasy and thinking? Why?

_____

_____

_____

Do you find you are never satisfied with your latest sexual fantasy—you want more or better?

_____

_____

_____

Have you hurt yourself by engaging in sexual fantasy or thinking—find yourself isolated, wasting too much time, disconnected from important relationships, or a source of harmful procrastination?

_____

_____

_____

Do you experience guilt or shame after having engaged in sexual fantasy and thinking? Describe.

_____

_____

_____

Have sexual fantasy and thinking affected your spiritual connection to God?

_____

_____

_____

Have you tried to end your sexual fantasy life? Why?

_____

_____

_____

Have you been successful? If yes, why? If not, why not?

_____

_____

_____

Do you find you are able to stop for a while but sooner or later you find yourself going back?

_____

_____

_____

Describe your favorite sexual fantasy?

_____

_____

_____

Why is this your favorite sexual fantasy?

_____

_____

_____

Have you noticed a connection between your favorite sexual fantasy and your desire to act out? Explain?

_____

_____

_____

Is there a connection between your favorite sexual fantasy and your specific acting out behavior?

_____

_____

_____

What connection does your favorite sexual fantasy have with your childhood abuse?

_____

_____

_____

If you ended your sexual fantasies and thinking, how would that change the frequency of your acting out? Explain.

_____

_____

_____

Do you want to end this behavior? Why?

_____

_____

_____

Sexual Encounters

Do you engage in sexual encounters outside of your marriage (or committed relationship)? For a non married man the question is: Have you had multiple relationships that frequently result in sexual relationships?

_____

_____

_____

How frequently do you engage in sexual encounters outside of your marriage (or committed relationship)? Why?

_____

_____

_____

What is the typical time lapse between sexual encounters outside of your marriage (or committed relationship)? Why?

_____

_____

_____

Who knows about your double life? How do they know?

_____

_____

_____

Are you fearful of being caught?

_____

_____

_____

What are the likely consequences of being caught?

_____

_____

_____

If you have been caught, what were the consequences?

_____

_____

_____

Do you find you are never satisfied with the current affair and you want someone new and exciting?

_____

_____

_____

Have you hurt someone in your life by sexual encounters outside of your marriage (or committed relationship)? Who? How has it affected your relationship with the person(s)?

_____

_____

_____

Do you experience guilt or shame after having engaged in an affair? Describe.

_____

_____

_____

Have sexual affairs affected your spiritual connection to God?

_____

_____

_____

Have you tried to stop having affairs? Why?

_____

_____

_____

Have you been successful? If yes, why? If not, why not?

_____

_____

_____

Do you find you are able to stop for a while but sooner or later you find yourself going back?

_____

_____

_____

Do you want to end this behavior? Why?

_____

_____

_____

Other Sexual Activities

Do you engage in phone sex, go to massage parlors, seek prostitution, seek same sex encounters, engage in exhibitionism, voyeurism, or other sexual activities?

_____

_____

_____

In which of these activities do you engage?

_____

_____

_____

When did your attraction to these activities begin?

_____

_____

_____

When did your attraction to these activities become a concern to you?

_____

_____

_____

How frequently do you engage in one or more of these activities? Why?

_____

_____

_____

What is the typical time lapse between engaging in one or more of these activities? Why?

_____

_____

_____

Do you lead a double life?

_____

_____

_____

Who knows about your double life? How do they know?

_____

_____

_____

Are you fearful of being caught?

_____

_____

_____

What are the likely consequences of being caught?

_____

_____

_____

If you have been caught, what were the consequences?

_____

_____

_____

Do you find you are never satisfied and you want more or better experiences?

_____

_____

_____

Have you hurt someone in your life by engaging in one or more of these activities? Who? How has it affected your relationship with the person(s)?

_____

_____

_____

Do you experience guilt or shame after having engaged in one or more of these activities? Describe.

_____

_____

_____

Have one or more of these activities affected your spiritual connection to God?

_____

_____

_____

Have you tried to stop this behavior? Why?

_____

_____

_____

Have you been successful? If yes, why? If not, why not?

_____

_____

_____

Do you find you are able to stop for a while but sooner or later you find yourself going back?

_____

_____

_____

Do you want to end this behavior? Why?

_____

_____

_____

Legality/Job Jeopardy

Does society consider any of your sexual behaviors illegal?

_____

_____

_____

When did your attraction to these activities begin?

_____

_____

_____

When did your attraction to these activities become a concern to you?

_____

_____

_____

Do you engage in Internet pornography or masturbation at your work site?

_____

_____

_____

Are you fearful of being caught?

_____

_____

_____

What are the likely consequences of being caught?

_____

_____

_____

If you have been caught, what were the consequences?

_____

_____

_____

Your story

Would you like to tell your story in your words? How would telling your story help you to get in touch with your concern(s)?

_____

_____

_____

_____

_____

_____

_____

_____

_____

_____

_____

What are the specific sexual behaviors that are of concern to you?

_____

_____

_____

When did your sexual behaviors begin?

_____

_____

_____

When did they become a concern to you?

_____

_____

_____

How frequently do you engage in these behaviors? Why?

_____

_____

_____

What is the typical time lapse between these behaviors? Why?

_____

_____

_____

Do you lead a double life?

_____

_____

_____

Who knows about your double life? How do they know?

_____

_____

_____

Are you fearful of being caught?

_____

_____

_____

What are the likely consequences of being caught?

_____

_____

_____

If you have been caught, what were the consequences?

_____

_____

_____

Do you find you are never satisfied and you want more or better experiences?

_____

_____

_____

Have you hurt someone in your life by these behaviors? Who? How has it affected your relationship with the person(s)?

_____

_____

_____

Do you experience guilt or shame after having engaged in these behaviors? Describe.

_____

_____

_____

Have these behaviors affected your spiritual connection to God?

_____

_____

_____

Have you tried to stop these behaviors? Why?

_____

_____

_____

Have you been successful? If yes, why? If not, why not?

_____

_____

_____

Do you find you are able to stop for a while but sooner or later you find yourself going back to these behaviors?

_____

_____

_____

Do you want to end these behaviors? Why?

_____

_____

_____

Sexual Addiction Questions

Now let's turn to questions that are relevant to all unwanted sexual behavior. Have your sexual practices become compulsive and unmanageable?

> What began as an occasional practice may increase to the point where you become powerless to stop. Do you find the need to compulsively repeat your sexual behaviors even after you promised yourself you would stop?

_____

_____

_____

Have you experienced life-damaging consequences as a result of your sexual behavior?

> Isolation is a primary consequence. Other consequences may include self-loathing, depression, anxiety, anger, despair, and pervasive feelings of hopelessness. The sexually-addicted man may find his relationships are damaged, particularly those with his family and his God. Shame and guilt become constant companions. What are the life damaging consequences you have experienced?

_____

_____

_____

Has your sexual behavior caused a change in your life focus?

> Sexual behavior becomes a primary motivator, and a primary need. Wanted or unwanted sexual behavior becomes so time consuming that it takes precedence over sleep, work, and healthy recreational activities. Paying for the cost of sex may take precedence over other family living expenses. Obtaining sexual gratification becomes so energy consuming that it displaces day-to-day functions and pleasures. Has sexual activity become a primary motivator in your life?

_____

_____

_____

Is keeping your sexual behavior a secret very important to you?

> Secrecy is a hallmark of sexual addiction. A sexually-addicted man fears he will be judged a bad person—someone with a problem he no longer can control. The addict believes he is evil and he is alone in his degeneration. Has secrecy kept you bound to your sexual behavior?

_____

_____

_____

Do you fear giving up your sexual behavior?

> The sexually-addicted man has lived with his sexual behavior for many years. The thought of not having daily or frequent encounters of acting out sexually is paralyzing to many. Intellectually, the sexual addict realizes he needs to change his life, but he is emotionally bound to his long-term habit, his best friend. Is your friendship with your sexual behavior keeping you locked into repeating your behavior?

_____

_____

_____

Have you denied that you have a problem related to sexual behavior?

> Invariably, the man who engages in a pattern of repetitive unwanted sex will develop illogical thinking to justify his behavior. Frequently heard excuses include: "I am not hurting anybody," "I deserve a little happiness in my life," "I plan to quit but I am under stress now," "I have a much higher libido than others I know and I need this outlet," "I can control this when I want to, and I don't need help," "It only happens once in awhile," "How else am I going to relieve my tremendous sexual tension?" Addicted men actually believe their lies and avoid getting the help they need. What lies have you told yourself or others to justify continuing your sexual behavior? What excuses do use to continue your sexual behavior?

Lies I believe . . .

Lie # 1

_____

_____

Lie # 2

_____

_____

Lie # 3

_____

_____

Lie # 4

_____

_____

Lie # 5

_____

_____

Excuses I have bought into . . .

Excuse # 1

_____

_____

Excuse # 2

_____

_____

Excuse # 3

_____

_____

Excuse # 4

_____

_____

Excuse # 5

_____

_____

Am I Sexually Addicted?

The questions you answered in this chapter are intended to give you insight into your sexual practices. How you answered any particular question in not necessarily a definitive indicator to the question, "Am I sexually addicted?" However, if you acknowledge that you have tried to stop your sexual behavior and have not been able to do so, even when you wanted to, it is likely that professional help is needed.

Questions related to frequency and time lapses between repeating sexual behavior are helpful to determine your profile. Men who exhibit long lapses between their episodes of sexual behavior may be as sexually addicted as the man who has frequent practices. The only difference is the length of one's acting-out cycle.

What is important is your profile. If, after you answer the questions, you have the gut feeling that "not all is well," then it is time to explore getting help.

When you examine your life do you find sexual behaviors you would like to leave behind? Can you answer the question, "Am I sexually addicted?"

Yes, I am sexually addicted. Why?

_____

_____

_____

No, I am not sexually addicted? Why?

_____

_____

_____

Maybe I am sexually addicted and maybe I am not. I am not sure yet. Why?

_____

_____

_____

I have examined my unwanted sexual behaviors and determined what I want to change:

Change # 1

_____

_____

_____

_____

Change # 2

_____

_____

_____

_____

Change # 3

_____

_____

_____

_____

Change # 4

_____

_____

_____

Change # 5

_____

_____

_____

_____

Wanting to change your behavior is important. However, it is rare for a sexually addicted man to change his addictive behavior over the long term without help. One man prayed for twenty-five years for God to take away his sexual addiction. He was sure God would do that for him. He finally learned that God's way of helping him was to give him the insight he needed to do the work of recovery. A quick fix did not exist.

Your Summary

What key points did you learn about yourself from this chapter?

Key Point 1:

_____

_____

_____

Key Point 2:

_____

_____

_____

Key Point 3:

_____

_____

_____

Key Point 4:

_____

_____

_____

Key Point 5:

_____

_____

_____

Chapter Two

Highlights of the Origin of Sexual Addiction

The upcoming pages summarize the origin of sexual addiction to help you to understand why you became sexually addicted, the topic of the next chapter. This information is from the book, *Recovery from Sexual Addiction: A Man's Guide*, a companion text to this workbook

Age-Inappropriate Exposure to Sexual Behavior or Material

A young child cannot be exposed to sexual behavior or material without consequences. A child does not have the life experiences to put such an event into perspective. Our sexuality begins very early in life and nature intends it to evolve as we age. It is normal for a young child to touch his genitals. It is not normal for a person other than a loving care giver to touch a child. A child instinctively knows the difference.

A child also instinctively knows that pornographic material is not part of his normal environment. Such exposure is traumatic to a child. For many, it is a trauma that they will remember for the rest of their lives. If parents do not normalize the event by putting it into perspective for the child, it may be a beginning factor which will lead to sexual addiction later in life.

Family Environment and Structure

Most sexually-addicted men come from a family environment that did not meet their childhood needs for affection or emotional support. Often children who live in dysfunctional families feel a sense of abandonment by their parents. The parents simply were not there for the child in a way that led to feelings of self-confidence and love. The child felt isolated from his parents and often his siblings.

When a child feels isolated and detached from his parents, he is unable to go to his parents with the confidence that they will love him when something bad happens. For most young children who are exposed to age-inappropriate behavior or material, instinct tells them that something bad has happened. If the child fears his parents' reaction to learning what happened, he will not confide in them. A lack of disclosure can be tragic. This is the very time that a child needs his parents most. It is critical that parents are called upon to explain to the child that his exposure was not his fault, and that, as a child he could not be responsible. Parental guidance is needed to explain that the normal body reaction to sexual touch or material—arousal—is not bad. It is normal at the proper time and circumstances. A traumatized child needs to know he is loved unconditionally and this bad event does not change his parent's love.

When a child believes he cannot trust his parents to love him at the time of exposure to age-inappropriate behavior or material, he may withdraw into himself and become even more isolated. He now has a huge troubling secret that he believes he cannot share. Many children begin to blame themselves for the event, even when all the logical signs point elsewhere. The child is often permanently damaged.

Most men who are sexually addicted did not have a close relationship with their father. While the child may have experienced emotional support from his mother, the lack of emotional support from the child's father plays a pivotal role in future addiction. The lack of emotional nourishment from the father seems to create the state of isolation necessary for the child to feel the need to self-mediate his feelings of emotional abandonment.

Some children who are exposed to unwanted sexual material or acts do not go on to have difficulty with adult sexual addiction. A child who is emotionally connected to his parents, particularly his father, doesn't find sexual stimulation necessary to enjoy life. An emotionally connected child who is exposed to age-inappropriate sexual material or behavior, who is able to relate the experience to his father, and whose father is able to respond in a nonjudgmental loving way, does not become sexually addicted.

Arousal

Arousal is the normal consequence of sexual stimulation—it is how God made us. Babies engage in self-stimulation. Doing so is the normal process of a self-discovery and learning the response to touch. But for a child who is introduced to sexual material or sex acts, the arousal is out of the norm. A child instinctively knows what normal stimulation is and realizes that the arousal he is experiencing is abnormal.

One of the reasons is intensity. When a child is first stimulated by sexual material or through the acts of another person, the intensity of the arousal is greater than normal self-stimulation. The child feels flooded with the new feelings. For the first time the brain is encoding the intensity of the feelings, and that encoding may remain for a life time. Do you remember the first time you were stimulated by sexual material or through the acts of another person? Do you remember the what, when, where and whom? How come you remember that experience with such clarity and not what you had for dinner on your birthday that year, which was another special occasion? The event was encoded in your brain. It was one of the defining moments of your life. The relationship between the child and parent is critical in defusing the intensity of the event.

While you may have felt other emotions, your brain remembers the chemical flow, the arousal feelings. Drug addicts who use cocaine tell researchers that the first high on cocaine is the best they have ever experienced. Many report that their continued use is an attempt to recreate the first high. Likewise, without realizing it, many sexually-addicted men try to recreate their first experience. For many, the sexual activity in which they engage as an adult has similar characteristics to sexual stimulus and arousal experienced in early childhood. For example, a child introduced to pornography may continue to be drawn to pornography as an adult. A child who is sexually abused is more likely to abuse other children in adulthood than a person who was not abused as a child.

Feelings of Shame, Guilt, and Depression

Shame and guilt are not the same. A man feels guilty when he knows he has done something wrong. Feelings of guilt can motivate a man to improve or change his behavior. Feelings of guilt emanate from his conscience talking to him.

On the other hand, a shamed man feels something is intrinsically wrong with him. A man who feels there is something wrong with him never enters into a loving and intimate relationship. Shame begets loneliness and contributes to a sense of sadness and depressed mood. He finds relief from his loneliness and depressed mood through sexual stimulation. The cycle becomes repetitive and compulsive. Negative feelings feed the need to feel good and act out sexually, which in turn cause feelings of shame and negativity and the cycle begins anew. No matter how many orgasms an addict experiences, he never escapes his shame. His depressed mood is only temporarily altered by orgasm.

For many men, the level of depression is not full blown but low grade. Low-grade depression differs from full depression only to the degree of the impact on one's daily functioning. For example, a fully depressed man may be unable to sleep properly, to eat, or to concentrate on the business at hand. Conversely, a man suffering low-grade depression functions each day but thinks he is missing the joys of life, feels tired much of the time, and finds living a burden. Such a person wakes up and says "Oh God, just another day," instead of "Good God, thanks for another day." This state of malaise goes on for years. It becomes painful and the prospect of escape through sex is inviting. Sex becomes a way of self-medicating the pain of life.

When a child is first sexually aroused by age-inappropriate behavior or material, he knows his new feelings are different. He knows what has happened occurred in a secretive environment. He may be told or understand he is not to tell. He knows it was wrong. He may feel guilt but, what is more important, the mind of a child is programmed to feel that he is bad, that something is terribly wrong with him. A child's sense of shame is set on fire by age-inappropriate sexual events. So much so that the feeling of shame, "I am defective," often stays with him for many years to come.

Learned Models in Childhood

Do you ever look in the mirror and see your dad? Do you see yourself repeating behaviors you once witnessed as a child? The answer is that behavior taught in childhood is often repeated in adulthood, even behavior that is despised by the child. So too, unwanted sexual behavior from childhood becomes unwanted sexual behavior in adulthood. Early childhood attachment to pornography is often repeated in adulthood. Abused children may abuse as adults. Children exposed to parental adulterous affairs, may engage in affairs as adults. In fact, a high percent of sexually-addicted men come from families where other addictions were present. If you are looking for the link to the type of unwanted sexual behavior that is giving you a problem today, look back into your childhood. You are likely to find the trail.

Your Summary

What key points did you learn about yourself from this chapter?

Key Point 1:

_____

_____

_____

Key Point 2:

_____

_____

_____

Key Point 3:

_____

_____

_____

Key Point 4:

_____

_____

_____

Key Point 5:

_____

_____

_____

Chapter Three

Why Did I Become Sexually Addicted?

Some modern day moralists say men choose to be sexually addicted, that is, to repeatedly engage in certain sexual acts. It constitutes a life choice to accept addiction. On the other hand, many experts believe that for the great majority of sexually-addicted men, the factors which led to addiction occurred long before the man was intellectually or emotionally capable of making a reasoned choice.

In this chapter we will explore the events that form the foundation or the "roots" for sexual addiction for a vast majority of men. They include:

- As a boy he was exposed to age-inappropriate sexual material or behavior.

- He was raised in a family environment in which his father was not capable of providing emotional nourishment to him.

- He experienced pleasurable arousal when he was exposed to age-inappropriate sexual material or behavior.

- Subsequent to exposure to age-inappropriate sexual material or behavior, he experienced feelings of shame, guilt, and isolation.

- Exposure to age-inappropriate sexual material or behavior occurred in secret and he did not feel safe in telling his parents.

- As a boy he began to repeat the activity or similar activity as the original exposure to age-inappropriate sexual material or behavior.

- As he grew into his teenage years, he repeated inappropriate sexual behavior.

- In adulthood inappropriate sexual behavior continued as a strong focus.

We will refer to these events as catalytic stories because they form the foundation for adult addiction. For a small proportion of sexually-addicted men the catalytic event was a function of a sexually sterile home environment. The home environment tolerated no discussion of sexual matters and, as a result, the child became like a sealed vacuum tube. At the time the young man left home or went away to college, the vacuum seal was broken and he inhaled sexuality. For these men, the catalytic event that forms the foundation for their adult sexual addiction occurred in their late teens or early twenties. If this applies to you, skip to page 45.

Sexual Addiction Often Begins in Childhood

If you are like most sexually-addicted men your addiction began in childhood, long before you understood what was happening. It occurred before you consciously understood what was happening to you. The following story contains common themes about the beginning of sexual addiction. See if you can identify them as you read this story.

Mark's story

Mark recalls being fondled by his teenage brother, Todd, when he was about six years old. He recalls the first time it happened. His brother was babysitting him and they were in his brother's bedroom sitting on Todd's bed. It was a treat to be in Todd's bedroom because normally Todd did not allow him into his room. To this day, he remembers Todd's bedspread and curtains had matching red and green plaid patterns.

Todd had several magazines hidden away in a drawer. He showed one of the magazines to Mark. He looked at the magazine picture and remembered wondering why someone would have their picture taken without their clothes on. He remembers Todd telling him he wanted to show him something that felt good. His brother took his pants down and touched him. Mark remembers feeling very confused because while being touched felt good—he liked the feeling—he also felt this was something they shouldn't be doing. He felt they were being bad.

Their parents came home early and Todd pulled Mark's pants up quickly and told him not to tell his parents. He wanted to tell his dad but was afraid his dad would be angry with him. He remembers his father often yelled at the boys, particularly after he had been drinking which was often. As Mark grew older, he found stimulating magazines similar to those his brother showed him and he engaged in sex play with younger children in the neighborhood. Mark did not have many friends and felt more comfortable in the company of younger children.

As an adult, Mark is sexually addicted. Let's examine the foundation of Mark's adult sexual addiction.

At what age was Mark introduced into age-inappropriate sexual material or behavior? Why was it age-inappropriate?

_____

_____

_____

What was Todd's age when he introduced Mark to inappropriate sexual material and behavior?

_____

_____

_____

Was Todd an age-appropriate companion for Mark? As such, what power did Todd have over Mark? Why does Todd's power make a difference?

_____

_____

_____

Describe the environment in which the catalytic event occurred? Why was secrecy important?

_____

_____

_____

What kind of a relationship did Mark have with his father?

_____

_____

_____

Why did Mark not feel comfortable telling his father what had happened?

_____

_____

_____

What feelings did Mark remember from his first exposure to pornography and molestation? Arousal feelings? Shame or guilt feelings?

_____

_____

_____

Do you see any indications that Mark was isolated from his peers?

_____

_____

_____

What behavior(s) did Mark begin to repeat as he grew older?

_____

_____

_____

What sexual behavior(s) do you project Mark engaged in as an adult?

_____

_____

_____

Your story

Mark's story is reasonably clear. Your catalytic story may or may not be as clear. For some men, it is a challenge to remember early exposure to age-inappropriate sexual material or behavior. It is common for these memories to be repressed or forgotten. It may take you some time to remember. For other men, the experience is as fresh as what happened yesterday.

The first retrieved memory may or may not be the addict's catalyst for his addiction. Some men remember their primary catalytic story later during therapy. Men often find the memory of their catalytic story causes pain and may be embarrassing. A child often blames himself for something he perceives to be wrong or bad. This may be particularly so if the man experienced considerable erotic pleasure.

Finally, some have difficulty recalling their catalytic story because they perceived what happened was normal. The event may have happened frequently or was perpetrated by a family member who the boy believed could not do something wrong or bad. For example, Billy was bathed by his mother each evening until age twelve. His mother took particular care to wash Billy's genitals. At times Billy got aroused. Billy had no other model of life to tell him that his mother's behavior was not normal.

For most men their story of exposure to age-inappropriate sexual material or behavior occurred between the ages of four and thirteen. It is possible your abuse took place earlier than age four but a child younger than four usually does not have the vocabulary or mental maturity to formulate a story to which he can relate later in life. However, a child does have feelings related to abuse which occurred before age four.

Sex play between children of the same age is normally not a catalytic event unless there is a notable difference in maturity between the children or the sex knowledge of one of the children is far more advanced than the other child. In other words, a catalytic event usually involves a differential in power.

Be patient with yourself as you recall your catalytic story.

At what age were you introduced to age-inappropriate sexual material or behavior? Why was it age-inappropriate?

_____

_____

How clearly do you remember the surroundings? Take a few minutes and record the surroundings. Where did it happen? What are the images and sounds you remember? Who else was there? What was your breathing like? What smells can you remember? Was there an atmosphere of secrecy?

_____

_____

_____

_____

_____

How old was the person and what was the relationship you had to the person who introduced you to age-inappropriate sexual material and behavior?

_____

_____

_____

Was this person an age-appropriate companion for you? As such, what power did the person have over you? Why did the person's power make a difference? What would have happened differently if the person did not have power over you?

_____

_____

_____

What kind of a relationship did you have with your father? Were you emotionally connected with your father? Were you emotionally connected with your peers?

_____

_____

_____

Did you feel comfortable telling your parents what had happened? Why? Did you tell anyone else?

_____

_____

_____

What feelings do you remember from your first exposure to age-inappropriate material and behavior? Were you excited, afraid, curious? Did you have mixed feelings?

_____

_____

_____

Did you have feelings of arousal? Was your body response physical or mental or both?

_____

_____

_____

Do you remember having feelings of being bad, shame, or guilt? Describe each.

_____

_____

_____

What are you feeling at this moment as you remember your catalytic event? Fear, shame, guilt, arousal, sadness, curiosity, confusion, numbness?

_____

_____

_____

Why do you think you are having these feelings as you remember your catalytic event?

_____

_____

_____

What behavior(s) did you begin to repeat as you grew older?

_____

_____

_____

What sexual behavior(s) have you brought into adulthood that began when you were a child?

_____

_____

_____

For Some Sexual Addiction Has its Origin in Late Teen Years or Early Twenties

Perhaps for you and one in ten men who become sexually addicted, the addiction had its origin in late teen years or early twenties. See if the following fits you. You grew up in a sexually sterile environment. Nothing sexual was ever mentioned or discussed in your home. Your parents and your siblings were always fully clothed, childhood sleepovers were not allowed. (In some cases, the child was home schooled.) You were isolated from life's normal educational events that provided for a healthy understanding of sexuality. This environment created a vacuum of sexual information and experience. The vacuum imploded once you left the family environment. When you experienced sexual stimulation for the first time in your late teens or early twenties, it caused your systems to go into overload, and, in turn, made sexual stimulation and orgasm exceptionally pleasurable and desirable. Compulsive repetition of the pleasurable experience turned into sex addiction.

Joshua's story—an alternative story

Joshua was raised in a highly disciplined family. From an early age he knew he was better off if he was seen and not heard. His brothers and sisters were very obedient to his parent's wishes. All members of the family had chores to begin and end the day. While the family dined together, a common theme at the family table was father's commentary on what was wrong with the world, the government, and the neighbors. The only discussion allowed by father was a supporting story or agreement.

Joshua felt his family was special; they knew what was right and what was wrong. However, he felt his family didn't fit in at church for they often came home right after church rather than attend church functions. Outside of members of his family he had few friends. He was not allowed to associate with neighborhood children who were not home schooled like he and his siblings were. The family watched only educational TV channels. There was no discussion of anything sexual. He had no knowledge of the human reproductive system until he was fifteen. He found it very hard to believe what a neighbor boy told him. He could not believe his parents would do "that."

Joshua believed he was raised in a loving environment. He knew his parents loved him; otherwise, why would they beat him when he was in error?

Joshua joined the military when he was eighteen. He was stationed far from home. His new buddies thought it was funny when Joshua told them he had never dated or kissed a girl. They helped Joshua make up for lost time. Joshua went wild with his new feelings. Sex became his primary need.

Your story, an alternative story

If the roots of your sexual addition were not found in early childhood sexual exposure, relate how you were first exposed to sexuality.

_____

_____

_____

_____

_____

_____

_____

_____

What behavior(s) did you begin to repeat?

_____

_____

_____

Did you make a conscious choice to become sexually addicted? Explain

_____

_____

_____

What Did I learn from the Last Two Chapters?

Are you now able to answer the question, "Why did I become sexually addicted?"

Now that you have identified the roots of your sexual addiction, you are empowered with knowledge to put into perspective the feelings of shame and guilt you have carried for years. Throwing off the bonds of shame and guilt is an important recovery step. When you accept that you are not a bad person but a person caught up in a problem, you can stand up straight and face those you love and your God. You can ask for insight to guide you on your recovery journey.

Remember you bought into the foundation of sexual addiction long before you were capable of making a conscious choice to be addicted. You did not ask to be sexually addicted—it happened to you. It is time to give up the past shame and guilt you have carried into the present time.

The present time is when you can make a choice to give up the burden of what happened to you as a child. Society demands we take responsibility for our actions. While you were not responsible for the roots of your sexual addiction, you are responsible for what happens as you move forward over time.

Feel free to make a new choice—to free yourself of the bonds of the past.

Your Summary

What key points did you learn about yourself from this chapter?

Key Point 1:

_____

_____

_____

Key Point 2:

_____

_____

_____

Key Point 3:

_____

_____

_____

Key Point 4:

_____

_____

_____

Key Point 5:

_____

_____

_____

Chapter Four

Why Can't I Just Stop?

You now know why you became sexually addicted. You have taken an important step. Your next step is to learn more about why ending inappropriate sexual behavior is a challenge.

Chances are you have promised yourself many times you will stop your unwanted sexual behavior. Perhaps for short periods of time you have stopped, but invariably you give in to temptation and you return to old habits of acting out. So, why can't you just stop?

Altering the Brain and Forming a Habit

The reason you, and all sexually-addicted men, find it difficult to "just stop" is your brain has become conditioned to demand satisfaction. Your brain tells you it needs the chemical flow, the rush caused by sexual stimulation.

Have you ever talked to a runner who has experienced a "runner's high?" A "runner's high" is a state of euphoria which occurs when chemicals, namely endorphins, increase in the brain. Endorphins are produced by the pituitary gland and the hypothalamus during strenuous exercise. The word "endorphin" comes from endogenous, which means "produced within the body." Endorphins, in turn, are neurotransmitters that are chemically similar to morphine. Morphine, a chemical substance derived from opium, elevates mood and reduces pain.

The same high experienced by runners is experienced by swimmers, skiers, football players, and others. Athletes note the high is similar to the experience of orgasm. Thus, the link is endorphins which are produced during exercise and orgasm. The athlete goes to considerable effort to achieve the high but the addicted man needs to go no further than stimulation. In fact, the high experienced from sexual stimulation and an orgasm is even more intense than a high experienced by the athlete because of the compressed time frame in which an orgasm takes place. Drug addicts pursue the same high. For the sexually-addicted man, sexual stimulation has become his drug of choice.

Take a few minutes to consider the feelings you experience <u>leading up</u> to orgasm. Describe them:

_____

_____

_____

Now describe the feeling you experience <u>during</u> orgasm. What is the level of intensity you felt?

_____

_____

_____

The high from sexual stimulation, particularly when repeated often, alters the neural pathways in the brain. The brain becomes addicted to the flow of endorphins and demands repetition of the stimulation.

It is no wonder, then, that the brain finds it difficult to give up the high experienced through orgasm. Once the brain's neural pathways are altered, saying "no" to the endorphin flow is painful and may trigger withdrawal symptoms including depressed mood or anxiety.

The altered neural pathways are the foundation of habit. Habits are formed over time. The longer an activity is practiced, the more ingrained it becomes. The more ingrained a habit becomes, the more difficult it is to change the habit. Achieving gratification becomes the addict's number one need.

How about you? How long have you repeated your acting-out sexual activity?

  A. At what age did you begin to repeatedly act out sexually? _____
  B. If you continued to act out, how old are you now? _____

  Subtract line A from line B. _____ This is how long you have been working
  to make your acting-out sexual activity part of your life, a habit.

Can addictive habits be changed? Yes, many smokers have stopped smoking. For some it took many tries. For some, they are still trying. Unfortunately, giving up smoking compared to giving up sexual behavior is an insufficient comparison. The greater the perceived reward, the high, the rush, the orgasm, the more ingrained is the perceived need to repeat the behavior.

If you want to rid yourself of your sexual-addiction habit, what are some of the remedies that come to mind? What could you do?

I could # 1

_____

_____

I could # 2

_____

_____

I could # 3

_____

_____

I could # 4

_____

_____

Perhaps you recorded such things as:

- I could put an Internet blocker on my computer.

- I could regularly attend a Twelve Step program.

- I could engage in individual or group sexual-addiction counseling.

- I could pray more.

- I could ask my wife to help me.

- I can read more to find out what I could do.

There are many actions a sexually-addicted man can do to reverse his acting-out behavior. You have already begun. For most men, the first step in the recovery process is to admit he has a problem which he cannot control. Hopefully you have recognized your behavior is out of control. The second most important change is to quit living in shame and guilt. Hopefully you have realized that shame and guilt are toxic to recovery. Later on in this workbook, other important steps will be addressed. For now, we need to turn back to addressing why it is difficult to stop acting out sexually. When you understand the enemy, you become empowered to reject its advances.

Sexual Fantasies

Just as a combustion engine cannot run very long without oil, many sexually-addicted men need a lubricating entity to continue acting out. For these men, sexual fantasies are the lubricant for acting out. If a man's brain is not stimulated, he will not achieve orgasm. The reality for most men, and in particular for the sexually-addicted man, is that his most powerful sexual organ is his brain and not his genitals. The endorphin flow begins as a man engages in sexual fantasy or sexual thinking.

The material to generate sexual fantasy is found everywhere for the sexually-addicted man. He finds it on the Internet, in the people walking down a street or sitting in a restaurant, in an image in a magazine, and, yes, even in a church. The sexually-addicted man has a fine-tuned filter in his head through which all visual images are processed for their sexual content. Some men focus on body parts while others focus on movement, facial expressions, or perceived come-ons. The sexually-addicted man either processes his sexual thinking in the present moment or stores the content away in the file cabinet in his brain to be incorporated into sexual fantasy at a later time.

For you, what are the sources and content of your sexual thinking and fantasies?

What are the multiple sources you use to begin sexual thinking and fantasy? Examples include Internet, magazines, on the way to work, the "file cabinet" in your brain. Describe each source and why it is a source for you.

Source # 1

_____

_____

Source # 2

_____

_____

Source # 3

_____

_____

Source # 4

_____

_____

Source # 5

_____

_____

What is the content of your sexual thinking or fantasies? For example, "I fantasize being seduced by "...."

My sexual thinking or fantasy content # 1

_____

_____

_____

My sexual thinking or fantasy content # 2

_____

_____

_____

My sexual thinking or fantasy content # 3

_____

_____

_____

My sexual thinking or fantasy content # 4

_____

_____

_____

Refer back to your answers on pages 10-14.

When you choose to engage in sexual fantasies or thinking, what reality are you escaping?

_____

_____

_____

_____

How do you feel about giving up your sexual fantasies and thinking, your best friend? Are you ready to try?

_____

_____

_____

_____

Your Acting-Out Environment

Sexual stimulation does not occur in a vacuum. It takes place at locations and at selective times. The sexual act is associated with other people, objects (clothing, sex toys), moods, smells, and, at times, taste. These environmental factors remind the brain that pleasure is nearby.

Jude's story

Jude was addicted to pornography. He spent his evenings and many nighttime hours searching the Internet for stimulating images of large-breasted women. The search never ended. Jude knew he needed to end his search. It consumed his time and his energy. His performance at work suffered due to lack of sleep. He vowed to stop.

Jude's sexually acting-out environment was his computer. Even the thought of turning it on got his juices going. But he had vowed to stop. Unfortunately, Jude began to deceive himself. He told himself he had other reasons for going on his computer, checking e-mail, for example. Jude told himself he would just check his e-mail. However, Jude's brain knew by past experience the act of turning on the computer is the first step toward sexual pleasure. Once the e-mail is checked, Jude told himself he just needed to check some other sites for whatever reason. The process continues until Jude finds a link (by accident, so he tells himself) which takes him down the road to pornography and acting out. Jude is not going to achieve his vow until he makes a choice to change his acting-out environment.

Your story

Do environmental factors remind your brain that pleasure is nearby?

What environmental factors begin your sexual quest? For example, silk sheets, sex toys, phone call, cigarette smoke, the computer, alcohol, drugs. Describe each and why it is a source for you.

Environmental factor # 1

_____

_____

Environmental factor # 2

_____

_____

Environmental factor # 3

_____

_____

Environmental factor # 4

_____

_____

Environmental factor # 5

_____

_____

Acting-Out Ritual

In the second paragraph of Jude's story on page 55, we read several steps Jude went through before resuming his acting-out behavior. These steps are called the acting-out ritual. The initial steps of the addict's ritual generally are benign, in that they are not in themselves adverse behavior. However, the brain of the addict knows these benign behaviors lead to acting out and thus are toxic. For example, Jude turned on his computer. There's nothing intrinsically wrong with Jude turning on his computer. However, Jude's brain, over time, learned that turning on the computer is simply the first step in Jude's acting-out ritual. Once the addict has passed through the initial steps of his acting-out ritual, he no longer has the power to reverse the end result of acting out. It is almost as if the addict enters into a hypnotic state once he begins his acting-out ritual. He becomes powerless to stop.

Lies and excuses that the addict tells himself during his ritual are the lubricant for acting out. If Jude was a fly on the wall and he listened to his reasoning as he proceeded through his ritual, he would be distressed. He would recognize his reasoning as fallacious and his excuses unbelievable. The addicted man in the throes of his ritual believes his own lies and excuses because they take him where he wants to go.

The acting-out ritual is one more element that makes it difficult for the addict to change his behavior. It is particularly so because the ritual begins with benign behaviors. The addict, after he has acted out again, will say to himself, I don't know how I got here because all I planned to do was check my e-mail. In his heart he would like to believe checking e-mail was all he planned to do. Unfortunately, the pull toward acting out is so strong, the addict does not learn from past failures. He repeats his ritual steps each time he acts out.

Sexually-addicted men usually have multiple acting-out rituals. Since addicted men do not learn by experience, it is important for them to get in touch with their various acting-out rituals. If the addicted man can learn to recognize the benign steps as toxic, he can empower himself to reject the ritual early in the ritual.

Tom's acting-out ritual

Tom engages in prostitution. Rituals are often connected to places, things, or activities. For example, Tom knew the location of every prostitution parlor in his city. Tom added another difficulty to his addiction. Tom only acted out about every six months. As such, a couple months after each sexual episode he convinces himself he does not have a problem. He is also oblivious to his acting-out ritual.

Let's examine Tom's acting-out ritual.

Tom's Acting-Out Ritual	Tom's Reasoning
Tom congratulates himself for having five months of sobriety	"I'm not a sexually-addicted man. I can control my behaviors. I have been sexually sober for five months."
Tom picks up a local newspaper	"It's been awhile since I've read the local newspaper; I wonder what I have missed."
Tom just happens to stumble over the section of the paper that includes personals and other relevant advertising	"I'm just checking to see what's new. I have no intention of giving up my five months of sobriety."
Tom sees a new ad.	"I am surprised to find something new, but it does not interest me."
Tom calls the number and learns what was being offered.	"I'm just checking this new place out. Perhaps I can be of help to another man by warning him about this place."
On Wednesday, Tom leaves work early to pick up software he ordered from a dealer across town.	"I know the place I called is close by to where I'm going, but I'll take a different route."
Tom finds himself parked near the new place.	"I can walk to the software dealer from here."
Tom finds himself at the front door of the new place.	"Since I am here, I will just check out the ladies. I will not go any further than that."
Tom talks to a very attractive woman.	"Where were these beautiful ladies when I was young? It is really fun to talk to an intelligent woman"
Tom pays for sex.	"I deserve a little pleasure in my dull life."

These are the steps Tom goes through before he acts out. These steps are called Tom's acting-out ritual. These are the lies, excuses, and justifications Tom uses to precede from step to step in his acting-out ritual.

For some men, the acting-out ritual is very short. For Joe, it can be summed up in one line. As Joe awakens in the morning he says to himself, I know I shouldn't masturbate, but I want to. For most men, the acting-out ritual is longer. For men who are trying to stop acting-out behavior, their acting-out ritual is replete with delusions to convince themselves they are not going where they know they are going.

Your acting-out rituals

Take time to identify and record your acting-out rituals. Most men have multiple acting-out rituals. The following pages provide space to record two of your acting-out rituals. Make them as detailed as possible.

As Tom did, record each step you go through before you act out; this is your acting-out ritual. After each step, record your reasoning; this is your self-talk. Pay particular attention to your reasoning; these are the lies you tell yourself and the excuses you use to justify your behavior.

This may be the most important work you do to help yourself understand why it is difficult for you to stop your acting-out behavior.

Your Acting-Out Ritual # 1	Your Reasoning
Step # 1	Reasoning # 1
Step # 2	Reasoning # 2
Step # 3	Reasoning # 3
Step # 4	Reasoning # 4
Step # 5	Reasoning # 5
Step # 6	Reasoning # 6
Step # 7	Reasoning # 7
Step # 8	Reasoning # 8
Step # 9	Reasoning # 9
Step # 10	Reasoning # 10

Your Acting-Out Ritual # 2	Your Reasoning
Step # 1	Reasoning # 1
Step # 2	Reasoning # 2
Step # 3	Reasoning # 3
Step # 4	Reasoning # 4
Step # 5	Reasoning # 5
Step # 6	Reasoning # 6
Step # 7	Reasoning # 7
Step # 8	Reasoning # 8
Step # 9	Reasoning # 9
Step # 10	Reasoning # 10

Sex-Addiction Cycle

It is time to see how all the impediments to ending addiction fit together. In fact, there is a paradigm which demonstrates how sequential factors make it difficult to stop acting-out behavior. It is called the Sex-Addiction Cycle.

In your mind, picture a circle like the face of a clock. On the top of the circle are conditions (depressed mood, negative thinking, pity party, etc.), that begin your acting-out cycle. At 3 o'clock are the factors (sexual thinking, fantasy, and environmental elements) that foster a build-up to acting out. At 6 o'clock is your acting-out ritual(s) with accompanying feelings of excitement and passion that lead you down the path to orgasm. At 9 o'clock are the shame and guilt you experience after acting out. Also at 9 o'clock are the promises you make to yourself to quit or to justify that acting out was not all bad. You return to 12 o'clock and it is only a matter of time before you repeat the cycle. In short, there is the beginning thought process, a build-up, the act, the let down, and a return to the beginning.

Below are the sequential steps or phases experienced by most sexually-addicted men. Within each phase the addict will engage in a thought process which leads him on. The time an addict takes to repeat the cycle can vary from minutes to months. A compulsive masturbator may act out five or more times a day, whereas a man involved in affairs may act out only when circumstances permit.

Note: Pay particular attention to the initial phase of your acting-out cycle. Men often find, in due course, when they become aware they are experiencing the life condition that begins their acting-out cycle, they can empower themselves to alter that particular life condition and thus forego acting out. Awareness leads to choices. For example, the life condition that begins John's acting-out cycle is low-grade depression. Now, when he recognizes he is experiencing depressed mood, he chooses to go to the gym. John has found that exercise brings him out of his depressed mood. John has taken an important step toward recovering from his sexual addiction.

Initial phase—Life Condition

On the left side of the table below are examples of life conditions in which the addicted man finds himself at the beginning of his sex addition cycle. Each condition is some form of negativity that exists in his life. You may or may not identify with one or more of the examples. On the right side of the table, note your understanding of the condition(s).

Victim posture. In my belief system, I am a victim in this world and not responsible for my behavior. In a new situation, I look for ways I will be hurt. I may not even know I look to be a victim. I have poor boundaries—people take advantage of me. **Low-grade depression.** Life for me is an existence; I often think life is passing me by. Except when acting out, I am rarely happy and I never feel joy. **Anticipated rejection.** I create situations in which someone else can reject me. I hold people at a distance. I can't let people know my real self—I know they will not love me. **Social isolation.** I live behind a mask of respectability but underneath my mask is my real self. I simply cannot let anyone in. If I did, they would see that I am really a bad person. I have few or no real friends. No one really knows who I am. **Emotional isolation.** I am not in touch with mine or other people's feelings. I don't understand that I hurt others. I don't understand my own feelings. For me, intimacy means sex.	**My life condition(s) when I begin my acting-out cycles is:** _____ _____ _____ _____ _____ _____ **Describe the reason(s) you think a life condition is the beginning of your sex-addiction cycle.** _____ _____ _____ _____ _____

Phase Two—Reaction to Life

On the left side of the table below are possible reaction(s) the addict uses to respond to his negative life conditions. Each reaction helps the addict to escape reality during his sex-addiction cycle. You may or may not identify with one or more of the examples. Go back and review your entries related to sexual thinking, fantasies, and environmental factors you employ to propel yourself toward acting out. On the right side of the table, note your understanding of the reaction(s) you use during your sex-addiction cycle.

Escapism. Living life is just too boring. I feel like life is just one painful experience after another. I need to find ways of relieving my bad feelings. **Need fulfilling fantasy.** I don't know how to cope, so I daydream of a better life. I use fantasy to get temporary relief. **Sexual thinking and fantasy.** I use sexual thinking, fantasies or visual sexual stimulation to escape my pain. My next act is often the subject of my fantasies and my sexual thinking. My fantasy is my best friend; we see each other a lot. **Sexual materials.** I maintain a well-used stash of pornographic magazines and movies, websites, and sex toys. Whenever I feel lonely, tired, or angry, my stash is nearby to raise my mood. **Altered brain-habit.** I have acted out so many times I really don't need an external stimulus. I just act out every morning/evening. I just have an overwhelming sexual feeling to which I respond.	**My reaction(s) to my life condition(s) that propel me toward acting out are:** _____ _____ _____ _____ _____ _____ **Describe the reason(s) you think you choose these reactions during your sex-addiction cycle.** _____ _____ _____ _____

Phase Three—Acting Out

On the left side of the table below is your acting-out state. Go back and review your entries related to what were the consequences of altering your brain and forming a sex-addiction habit. On the right side of the table, note your acting-out ritual and the nature of how you act out.

	My acting-out ritual is:
Acting-out ritual. I mentally begin a ritual which leads me to act out. At times I play games with myself. Examples include: I tell myself I will just go a little way but not all the way but I go all the way. I go to my computer to check e-mail but not porn but I end up at a porn site. **Acting-out.** Sex is my most important need. I act out sexually even when I don't want to.	_____ _____ _____ _____ _____ _____ _____ _____ _____ _____ _____ _____ _____ _____

Phase Four—Reconciliation

On the left side of the table below are possible reaction(s) the addict experiences after acting out. Each reaction keeps the addicted man glued to his shame and guilt—even his excuses which would seem to relieve him of responsibility. Intuitively he knows such excuses are lies. He tells himself lies in order to deal with shame and guilt. Go back and review your entries related to shame and guilt. On the right side of the table, note the reaction(s) that you use after acting out.

Transitory guilt. I feel sorry and I am ashamed of myself. I fear being caught. My focus is on what is going to happen to me. I am unaware of how I hurt my family. My feeling of guilt is short-lived. **Reconstruction.** I present outwardly as a good guy. I seek forgiveness at church. I am never going to do it again. I am going to make it right. I conceal my act. **Mistaken beliefs.** I didn't hurt anybody. I deserve some pleasure in life. **Thinking errors.** I can control my behavior if I want to. I don't need any help. What do they know about my problem?	**What is your reaction(s) to acting out?** _____ _____ _____ _____ _____ **What are your shame and guilt outlets?** _____ _____ _____ _____ _____

Once completed, the addict returns to the initial phase and begins the cycle anew.

Your Summary

What key points did you learn about yourself from this chapter?

Key Point 1:

_____

_____

_____

Key Point 2:

_____

_____

_____

Key Point 3:

_____

_____

_____

Key Point 4:

_____

_____

_____

Key Point 5:

_____

_____

_____

Are You Discouraged?

After reading this chapter, are you discouraged? Perhaps you thought it would be relatively easy to rid yourself of unwanted sexual behavior. Unfortunately, for most men the journey takes a lifetime. The good news is many men have discovered how to live in recovery. In Chapter 7 we talk about hope—the ingredient to recovery.

Other conditions contribute to making it difficult for the sexually-addicted man to quit his acting-out behavior. The most important of which is living in a depressed mood. Most sexually-addicted men find life just bearable and rarely experience joy. Mental health professionals call this state Dysthymic Disorder or low-grade depression. Other conditions include living with anxiety and anger. The sexually-addicted man almost always is emotionally isolated from his peers. These conditions will be addressed in the next chapter.

Chapter Five

Role of Anger, Anxiety, Depression and Isolation in Sexual Addiction

Sexual addiction is like an iceberg. Above the surface is the addict's acting-out behavior. In order for an addict to recover, he must realize that the bulk of his addiction—and the very key to his recovery process—is in what lies beneath the surface. Below the surface are many conditions (anger, anxiety, depressed mood, and isolation) that accompany and contribute to sexual addiction. When the dysfunction beneath the surface is understood, choices become clearer, recovery becomes easier.

Why do sexually-addicted men also experience anger, anxiety, low-grade depression, and isolation? When the male child does not receive the emotional nourishment he needs, particularly from his father, the resulting condition creates a significant deficit in the psyche or a hole in the soul of the child. The hole in the soul becomes vulnerable to anger, anxiety, and depression. These factors are compounded by shame, and guilt which cause the child to become isolated. The child reaches out to sexual stimulation in place of supporting relationships and normal childhood development. When a child experiences isolation, that is, a distancing from parents, siblings, and peers, he begins to see the world as a frightening place. The world is no longer happy or safe.

An isolated child feels alone in the world. Because of his acting-out behavior, he often sees himself as a bad person. He sees his peers as popular, more talented in sports, or doing well in the world. On the other hand he wonders why it is he who goes back to sexual stimulation to feel okay. A child who grows up in a negative world may become an adult who is angry, anxious, and suffering from low-grade depression. He also brings his isolation into adulthood. He sees himself as a second-class citizen.

Let's examine each of these factors and see the role each has played in your life.

Childhood Emotional Nourishment

When asked, sexually-addicted men often say they had normal childhoods. They will talk about how their mothers did the best they could in often difficult circumstances. Almost universally they will talk about their fathers in the context of a distant relationship. Often, these men say the following things about their fathers.

- My father was not present in the family by choice; he left the home when I was young.

- My father was dominated by my mother to the extent of being emasculated.

- My father was a loner. I could never talk with him.

- My father was abusive physically, sexually, or mentally.

- My father was sexually addicted. I found his stash of pornographic magazines when I was young.

- My father was a workaholic.

- My father isolated himself from the family through sports, interests outside the home, or a hobby.

- My father was absent because of his addiction to drugs, alcohol, or sex.

Sexually-addicted men, more often than not, had fathers who were dysfunctional or had significant problems. It is common for sexual addiction to be passed down from generation to generation.

When challenged about his childhood, it may be difficult for the man to see how his relationship with his father was anything but normal because he has no other experience or family model to which he can compare his family. Yes, he remembers other fathers who were there for their children, but he considers those fathers to be above normal.

Ely's story

Ely was asked to talk about his relationship with his father.

"My dad was a very loving father to me and my brothers. He was there for us. I knew he loved me and my brothers because he beat us often, particularly when we didn't behave. I remember a couple times when I was beaten so badly that . . ."

Eventually Ely came to this conclusion, "My dad did love me, but not in the way I needed to be loved in order to be emotionally healthy." Ely's father did not provide Ely or his brothers with a safe and nourishing environment.

Let's see what your iceberg looks like below the surface.

Your family of origin

Your family relationships formed your outlook on life. You either thrived as a result of the love you received or floundered as a result of being starved for affirmation, support, and love.

What about your family? How would you describe your relationship with your mother?

_____

_____

_____

How would you describe the relationship between your mother and your father?

_____

_____

_____

Did you witness daily expressions of love and respect between your parents? If no, why do you think that was so?

_____

_____

_____

What kind of man was your father?

_____

_____

_____

Was your father present for the family? Was your father a workaholic? Did he isolate himself from the family through sports? Did he have time-consuming interests outside the home? Did he have a hobby or workshop in which he spent much time alone? Was he addicted to drugs, alcohol or sex? Was he abusive physically, sexually, or mentally? If so, write these answers down. Share your feelings, your pain.

_____

_____

_____

_____

_____

How would you describe your relationship with your father?

_____

_____

_____

If, as a child, you had a distant relationship with your father, what story did you tell yourself to explain your father's lack of attention or concern for you?

_____

_____

_____

If you had a distant relationship with your father, how do you describe the love between the two of you?

_____

_____

_____

At what age do you remember your father saying, "I love you?"

_____

_____

_____   _____

Can you remember examples of feeling abandoned by your father?

_____

_____

_____

Childhood Messages

Parents, teachers, and other people send messages to the child. These messages may be ego enhancing. For example, a child who is tucked into bed each evening and told by his parents how much he is loved, is likely to take the message of love into adulthood. On the other hand, parents may send messages that harm the ego of the child. If a parent continually tells a child he is a bad boy when something goes awry, the message he may internalize is that he is bad or even evil.

Some common messages sent by dysfunctional parents are:

- It is not safe to express your feelings.

- We will love you only if you do well in school or sports.

- There is no time for play around here. You need to fix dinner and take care of your siblings.

- You are a failure!

- Your opinion doesn't count in this house. I will tell you what to think!

- You need to be the man of the house.

- Bs on your report card are not good enough. You can do better.

- You will never measure up to our expectations.

- I will give you something to cry about.

- You are bad just like your father.

- You couldn't possibly amount to anything.

- Children are to be seen, not heard.

- Why can't you be like your older siblings?

Each of these statements is harsh and negative. Each expresses a judgment. The child learns that love for him is conditional. He is not a person of worth. Life is negative. Negative feelings lead to negative judgments about self. If a child does not feel the joy of being loved unconditionally, chances are he will respond to life on the opposite side of the spectrum—with anger and depressed mood.

Were you blessed by loving messages from your parents? Were you devalued by critical messages from your parents? What are some of the messages you received?

Message 1

_____

_____

Message 2

_____

_____

Message 3

_____

_____

Message 4

_____

_____

Message 5

_____

_____

Message 6

_____

_____

Message 7

_____

_____

How did these messages impact your belief about yourself?

_____

_____

_____

Did any of these messages contribute to your feeling of isolation from your parents?

_____

_____

_____

Of the messages you received, which ones contributed to a positive self-image? Of the messages, which ones contributed to a negative self-image?

Positive:

_____

_____

_____

Negative:

_____

_____

_____

As you answer these questions, what are your feelings in the present moment? Are you angry, sad, depressed, anxious, perplexed, numb, happy, or unhappy? Describe your feelings.

_____

_____

_____

_____

_____

_____

_____

As a child, were you emotionally nourished to the extent that you felt okay about yourself? If not, do you think your family environment played a role in you becoming a sexually-addicted man? How?

_____

_____

_____

Do you feel a lack of emotional nourishment in your adult relationships or in your marriage? Does a lack of emotional nourishment help to keep you addicted?

_____

_____

_____

Role of Anger

Anger can be exhibited in different ways. For example, anger can be active and is evident though fits of rage, yelling or screaming, destroying property, or attacking another person. Or anger can be passive and is evident through withdrawing from a conversation when you feel overwhelmed or unable to "control" the outcome of the discussion. Other expressions of anger include frequently engaging in criticism, becoming cynical in your evaluation of others, and making sarcastic remarks to appear superior over others.

What role does anger play in your life?

_____

_____

_____

As a child, do you remember expressions of anger in your family? Which members? Were you the recipient of anger?

_____

_____

_____

If you expressed anger, what was your parents' response?

_____

_____

_____

Do you remember anger causing problems in school, sports, or relationships? If so, share some examples.

_____

_____

_____

How did you express anger in your late teens?

_____

_____

_____

In the present time, do you often express anger? If so, how? Share two examples.

Example:

_____

_____

_____

Example:

_____

_____

_____

Are you angry at God? If so why? Are you angry at God for not removing your addiction? If so, share what you have shouted at God.

_____

_____

_____

_____

_____

_____

_____

Does anger play a role in keeping you isolated and addicted?

_____

_____

_____

_____

What is the relationship between your anger and acting out?

_____

_____

_____

_____

Paul Becker, LPC

Role of Anxiety

Anxiety is a state of emotional discomfort, one in which a person often feels a loss of the control to manage a situation or event.

Anxiety can be situational, for example, feeling very uncomfortable in social gatherings. It can be chronic, for example, making a person feel on the edge much of the time, sometimes for entire days. Anxiety can be sexual, for example, a tense feeling in your genital region that you believe will go away by masturbating.

What role does anxiety play in your life?

_____

_____

_____

Was anxiety a characteristic experienced by any member of your family? Which members?

_____

_____

_____

As a child, do you remember being anxious?

_____

_____

_____

What was your parents' response to your anxiety?

_____

_____

_____

Do you remember anxiety causing problems in school, sports, or relationships? If so, share some examples.

_____

_____

_____

How did you express anxiety in your late teens?

_____

_____

_____

Do you consider yourself to be an anxious person in the present time? If so, how?

_____

_____

_____

Did you or do you masturbate to relieve anxiety?

_____

_____

_____

As an adult, do you frequently experience sexual anxiety or a tense feeling in your genital region that you believe will go away by masturbating? Describe a typical situation. How frequently do you experience sexual anxiety?

_____

_____

_____

_____

_____

As an adult, do you take medication to mitigate anxiety symptoms? If so, describe the events around the diagnosis that lead to your taking medication.

_____

_____

_____

Roles of Depressed Mood

Perhaps the most debilitating condition a sexually-addicted man carries through life is a propensity to live in a depressed mood. Living in a depressed mood is an almost universal characteristic of sexually-addicted men. A man who masturbates to relieve chronic anxiety may not necessarily live in a depressed mood.

A depressed mood is a significant part of the addicted man's below-the-surface iceberg. It is hard for an addicted man to see and appreciate beauty, wholesome love, joy, or many other uplifting attributes normal to healthy people. Instead, the focus is on what is going wrong in life, rather than what is going right. It is a condition which fosters acting out.

It is not known whether isolation causes depression or depression causes isolation, but the two conditions frequently co-exist. Both tendencies begin in childhood for the sexually-addicted man. After having been exposed to sexual material or behavior and having found arousal to be a pleasurable feeling, the child begins to return to these behaviors for relief from the detachment he feels from parents and peers. Once he begins to engage in sexual behavior on a frequent basis, the feelings of shame and guilt convince him that he is both bad and unusual. The tangled web of dysfunction results in a chronically depressed mood.

Chronic depressed mood

The mental health community calls chronically depressed mood a Dysthymic Disorder. Dysthymia is characterized as a depressed mood lasting at least two years during which the person experiences a continuous feeling of malaise. (American Psychiatric Association, 2000) Not much in life is going great but, at the same time, one is not so deeply depressed that he cannot function. Perhaps another appropriate descriptive term is low-grade depression. Those who experience low-grade depression often have low energy, low self-esteem, and a general feeling of hopelessness. Sexual addicts who are depressed do not feel good about themselves and are aware that they live behind a mask of respectability. They feel deep inside they are terribly flawed.

For most sexually-addicted men, a depressed mood accompanies awaking each morning. Life is simply not meeting expectations. One man said, "I got in a rut and then I furnished it!" When asked, the sexually-addicted man talks about unfulfilled relationships with parents, siblings, and, in particular, his spouse. He has few, if any, close friends. He feels lonely much of the time. He looks for more from life but does not seem to ever find it. He finds he procrastinates because he fears failure. Profound feelings of shame haunt him. The tone of his description of himself has elements of "poor me." Other men use the cliché, "Life is a bitch, and then you die."

What role does depressed mood play in your life?

Your chronic depressed mood

As you read the descriptions of chronic depressed mood, what comes to mind that defines your depressed mood?

Example:

_____

_____

Example:

_____

_____

Example:

_____

_____

Example:

_____

_____

Example:

_____

_____

Example:

_____

_____

Perhaps a visual tool will help to explain how low-grade depression relates to acting out. This visual tool is called: The **Addict's Life Scale**. This scale ranges from "0" to fifty in ten-point increments. Each benchmark on the scale correlates with a relative mood level. We will begin by defining a few terms.

- The euphoria experienced during orgasm is a fifty-point benchmark level.

- Normal functioning mood is at the forty-point benchmark level. It is the mood level of solid strength and energy. It is the "great to be alive" mood level.

- A bad day is at thirty-point benchmark level. Men who live at forty occasionally visit the thirty-point benchmark but do not live there.

- Low-grade depressed mood is at the twenty-point benchmark level. For most sexually-addicted men, it is the level of mood that accompanies daily life. Life is simply not meeting expectations.

- Full-scale depressed mood is at the ten-point benchmark level. This person finds it difficult to eat, sleep, and go about daily life.

- Unable to function is at the zero-point benchmark level. This person often requires institutionalization.

- See the book, *Recovery from Sexual Addiction: A Man's Guide*, for a full description of each benchmark mood level and for a discussion of **Addict's Life Scale**.

Addict's Life Scale

50—Acting-out mood. The feeling of euphoria one feels during the build-up and experience of an orgasm.

40—Normal Functioning Mood. The ideal mood level of a normally functioning adult. It is a, "great to be alive," mood level.

30—Bad Day Mood. A level to visit but not stay.

20—Low-grade Depressed Mood or Dysthymic Disorder. Where most addicts live life.

10—Full Scale Depressed Mood. The person barely functions.

0—Unable to Function Mood. The person is often institutionalized.

If there is an ideal mood level, it is represented by forty on the **Addict's Life Scale**. For the purposes illustrated here, it is a healthy level to which sexually-addicted men aspire but do not achieve.

At the fifty-point benchmark level, the acting-out level, an addict feels a sense of euphoria, a high, a rush. The orgasm is the end product, it is the goal, it is the relief from life's pain. His pain is so unacceptable he is willing to go for the short-term fix. He tells himself:

- I need this!

- I can't live without my fix.

- Life is a bear. I deserve this to be happy once in awhile.

- I earned it!

- Oh, the hell with it, I am going for it!

The key for the addict is to begin to change his life so that the forty-point benchmark level, the "great to be alive" mood level, becomes more of the norm than the twenty-point benchmark level, low-grade depressed mood. The differential between forty and fifty is only ten points. Men who make the effort to change how they live so as to experience frequent forty-point benchmark level, "great to be alive," feelings, find that a ten-point differential is not enough of a reward to offset the negative consequences of acting out.

Your life scale

How does the **Addict's Life Scale** apply to your life? At what benchmark mood level do you awaken each day? Do you know why you live at that level?

Take a few minutes to record your thoughts on the **Addict's Life Scale** below.

50—Acting-out mood. The feeling of euphoria one feels during the build-up and experience of an orgasm.

_____

_____

_____

40—Normal Functioning Mood. The ideal mood level of a normally functioning adult. It is a, "great to be alive," mood level.

_____

_____

_____

30—Bad Day Mood. A level to visit but not stay.

_____

_____

_____

20—Low-grade Depressed Mood or Dysthymic Disorder. Where most addicts live life.

_____

_____

_____

10—Full Scale Depressed Mood. The person barely functions.

_____

_____

_____

0—Unable to Function Mood. The person is often institutionalized.

_____

_____

_____

Next steps

Because thinking, feelings, behavior, and mood have been ingrained over many years, it is unlikely that most men will be able to live at the forty-point level all of the time, or even for most of each day. But it is possible to begin to consciously program in a level of forty-point behaviors that are mood lifting and sufficient enough to begin to change the addiction dance. It is possible to consciously choose to remodel one's rut.

Men who live at the twenty benchmark level are encouraged to select and engage in multiple forty benchmark level activities each week. Unfortunately, if forty benchmark level activities are not planned in advance, they will not happen. Men who live at twenty, simply don't think about "draining the swamp when they are up to their '. . .' in alligators." A man in therapy is encouraged to engage his partner in a "40 planning session" over the weekend. During the planning session they commit to paper such activities as:

Monday:	Go to the gym.
Tuesday:	Talk after dinner for 30 minutes.
Wednesday:	Go to the gym.
Thursday:	Take a walk together . . . include the children.
Friday:	Go out for a Pizza dinner . . . include the children but sit them at an adjacent booth.
Saturday:	Marital relations.
Sunday:	Engage in spiritual nourishment. Plan next week's forty benchmark level activities.

It is important to plan one or more marital relations in order to provide the addict with opportunities to delay gratification as opposed to acting out.

Role of Isolation

An isolated man is a lonely man. Loneliness is a breeding ground for depressed mood and a sad life. Inappropriate anger keeps the addict detached from people. Instead of drawing people to him, he distances himself using his anger responses. Anger keeps the sexually-addicted man isolated.

In childhood, isolation can take many forms. Some common examples heard are: I stayed to myself; I had a few friends but I was not as popular as I would have liked; I was frequently picked on by siblings or others; I spent a lot of my time in video games, TV, and individual activities; kids laughed at me; I found it difficult to share my concerns and feelings with my parents; I played or engaged in sex play with younger children; I found acceptance from the wrong crowd.

What role does isolation play in your life?

_____

_____

_____

Would you describe yourself as isolated as a prepubescent child (5-12), as a young teenager (13-15), as an older teenager (16 and up)?

_____

_____

_____

Were you always isolated from your family and peers or did it occur later on? What caused the change?

_____

_____

_____

Give a few examples of how you were isolated from parents, peers, or siblings.

Example:

_____

_____

_____

Example:

_____

_____

_____

What were your thoughts or feelings related to isolation? For example, I just felt I wasn't normal, I felt parents and teachers didn't understand me, I felt sad that I was not part of the "in" group.

_____

_____

_____

Are you isolated as an adult? Give several examples.

Example:

_____

_____

_____

Example:

_____

_____

_____

Did a lack of healthy emotional nourishment contribute to your isolation? Explain your understanding.

_____

_____

_____

Did exposure to age-inappropriate sexual material or behavior contribute to your isolation? Explain your understanding.

_____

_____

_____

As an adult, from whom are you isolated? What are your feelings related to being isolated from these people?

_____

_____

_____

Does isolation play a role in keeping you addicted?

_____

_____

_____

Your Summary

What key points did you learn about yourself from this chapter?

Key Point 1:

_____

_____

Key Point 2:

_____

_____

Key Point 3:

_____

_____

Key Point 4:

_____

_____

Key Point 5:

_____

_____

Keep in mind

Not every man who experienced a distant relationship with his father, was sexually abused or exposed to age-inappropriate material or behavior becomes sexually addicted as an adult. However, a high percentage of sexually-addicted men did experience a distant or nonexistent relationship with their fathers and were sexually abused or exposed to age-inappropriate material or behavior.

In addition, the majority of sexually-addicted men who experienced a distant or nonexistent relationship with their fathers and were sexually abused or exposed to age-inappropriate material or behavior also deal with anger, anxiety, isolation, and low-grade depression as an adult. Sexually-addicted men generally experience low-grade depression or anxiety but usually not both.

The underlying principle of sexual addiction is mood alteration. When a man engages in his acting-out ritual and subsequently acts out, his mood is temporarily lifted. He escapes his pain.

Chapter Six

Codependency

Clinical experience has shown that sexually-addicted men, when they marry, often marry into a codependent relationship. Codependency will affect the marriage and may affect the addict's recovery. Both partners may find it beneficial to examine their role in the marriage.

The term codependency was first coined in the Alcoholic Anonymous community. As it relates to sexual addiction, I define codependency as the propensity of marriage partners to look for happiness or the lack of contentment based on the behavior of the partner. In simpler terms, each partner expects the other partner to cause their happiness. Melody Beattie (1992), a well known author in the field of codependency defines codependency as:

> A codependent person is one who has let another person's behavior affect him
> or her, and who is obsessed with controlling that person's behavior.

For the sexually-addicted male, there is a clear road map to codependency. It is almost universal that the sexually-addicted man did not have a nourishing relationship with his father—and in some cases, with his mother, when his mother assumed the characteristics of the paternal role in the family. Again, the vast majority of sexually-addicted men grew up in a dysfunctional family, often abusive, and most often with parents who were codependent themselves. It is natural for the sexually-addicted man, when he seeks a partner, to find one who also experienced dysfunction and codependency in her family.

Perhaps, as you read the description of codependency you will find elements that relate to you.

Codependency in Marriages Where the Male Is Sexually Addicted

When a sexually-addicted man marries into a codependent relationship, his spouse often plays the role of the mother who feels responsible for fixing her child (husband)—a way of controlling him or making herself feel indispensable. Since the man likely did not learn good communication or parenting skills from his family of origin, he gives his spouse plenty of opportunities to tell him about his deficiencies. The addicted man plays the role of the damaged child who needs someone to chastise and fix him. The wife takes the superior position in the marriage and the addicted man takes the subordinate position. The marriage is unbalanced. Mutual respect and acceptance of one another on the basis of equality is absent. Unfortunately, the unbalanced marriage helps to keep the man steeped in his sexual addiction.

Interestingly, the spouse does not see herself in the superior position. She sees herself in the victim position. She sees herself as the recipient of her partner's broken promises to do better, his inability to show affection other than through sex, and his inability to communicate except through anger, etc.

She sees the man whom she thought she loved fail miserably as the husband she thought she married. She keeps trying to help (or fix) him because she craves the husband of her dreams.

Frequently, her family of origin was dysfunctional and did not provide her with the loving nourishment she needed to feel whole. She looked to marriage to fill the gaps in her life. She too is hurting in the marriage. Her need for the husband of her dreams is conditioned by her own insecurity, her own feelings of being abandoned, and her sorrow at not being connected to her husband. Although the above is not a universal characterization of the marriage relationships among all sexually-addicted men and their spouses, it is reality for many.

Neither partner is getting what they expected nor what they need from the marriage relationship. His isolation grows and he uses his addiction to medicate his pain of isolation. Her effort to help (or fix) her husband has the exact opposite of her intended effect and she grows more frustrated with his failures.

Who is to blame?

This chapter is not intended to assess blame on one or both partners. It merely conveys the reality that is found in many relationships involving a sexually-addicted person.

The Origin of Codependency Is Found in a Child's Dysfunctional Family

Parents of codependent children are often codependent themselves. The traits are handed down, that is, taught to each succeeding generation. The parents of the codependent children are ill equipped to provide emotional nourishment to their children. Instead, dysfunctional families abound in addiction, narcissism, and the inability to show love to their children. When parents are internally focused on their own problems, they are ill equipped to build healthy relationships with their children. They can't give what they don't have.

Children of Codependent Dysfunctional Families Have Ill-formed or Incomplete Personalities

Adult behavior, either intentionally or not, builds on the dysfunctional personality traits learned in the family of origin. Men from dysfunctional families often are deficient in their social skills and question their self-worth. Because of this low self-esteem, they often wonder if anyone really could love them. Nevertheless, distorted thinking leads them to equate sex with a feeling of being loved.

In Marriage, Codependency Fosters Pain and Negativity

Once married, men often repeat the cycle they began before marriage. They lack marriage skills and pursuits outside of the marriage bed further distanced them from providing the emotional nourishment their partner dearly needs.

Codependency Addressed

In a healthy marriage, partners see themselves neither in a superior position nor as the victim, but as equals. Each takes individual responsibility to grow in wisdom. The goal of the addict is to accept that he has a problem which he needs to commit to address. The wife's goal is to accept that she, too, has issues that she could address. Both need to support each other in a quest to become whole, and shun the paralyzing effects of shame.

In a codependent relationship, each partner's identity lies outside of the self. Each depends on the other to provide wholeness. Neither partner is independent in the relationship. For example, if you would like to change your partner's behavior, you are saying, "For me, happiness lies in how my partner can change, not on how I function independently." In a codependent relationship, both parties want to be in charge but neither party feels that they are, and yet, each party feels the other is in charge.

A visual picture of codependency relationship

Picture two elevators side by side: The male occupies one and his partner the other. When the partner's elevator is on the tenth floor, the male's elevator is in the basement. When the male's elevator is in the basement, he sees himself as the errant child and he looks up to his partner on the tenth floor and sees a scornful mother. He gives his partner the power to chastise, for he believes he deserves it, but he intensely resents her for doing so. His partner takes the power given to her and dutifully scolds and punishes. She is no longer the spouse, but has taken the role of the dysfunctional mother.

They ride their elevators to the opposite levels. His partner's elevator is now in the basement and he is on the tenth floor. His partner sees herself as the victim of his self-centeredness. She sees his behavior as willful, destructive to the marriage, and selfish. She sees him in a superior position—doing his own thing without regard to the consequences, particularly to the marriage. He supports her vision by continuing to put his sexual needs first.

They continue to ride their respective elevators, alternating between the basement and tenth floor. As they ride, they get more and more angry, and blame each other for their predicament.

What needs to change?

In simplistic terms, both would do well to ride their elevators to the fifth floor, get off, and face one another.

Ideally, he admits he is powerless to stop his behavior—it has become unmanageable.

His partner rejects the role of his mother. She tells him, "It is not my job to change you. That is your challenge." If so inclined, she can tell him, "If you would like a friendly ear while you are in therapy, I may agree to listen, but I am not willing to try to be your accountability partner or make suggestions."

She may choose to deal with the origins of her codependent behavior in individual or group therapy.

His fifth floor position is to thank his partner and to commit to counseling. His therapist will likely also recommend he attend one or multiple Twelve-Step programs on a regular basis.

What role does codependency play in your life?

_____

_____

_____

Do you recognize symptoms in your behavior? Give examples.

Example:

_____

_____

_____

Example:

_____

_____

_____

Example:

_____

_____

_____

Example:

_____

_____

_____

Do you recognize symptoms in your partner's behavior? Give examples.

Example:

_____

_____

_____

Example:

_____

_____

_____

Example:

_____

_____

_____

Example:

_____

_____

_____

Give a few examples of how you believe codependency keeps you stuck in sexual addiction.

Example:

_____

_____

_____

Example:

_____

_____

_____

Example:

_____

_____

_____

What do you believe needs to change?

_____

_____

_____

How would marriage counseling help you and your partner to address codependency?

_____

_____

_____

Chapter Seven

Is There Hope?

You have completed an extensive review of the human factors related to sexual addiction. You have examined the life conditions that bind sexually-addicted men to their addictions. The purpose of asking you to look inward is to see how you identify with the characteristics of sexually-addicted men. It is not to discourage you or to make recovery a formidable challenge. The premise is this: the more insight you have into the what, where, and why of sexual addiction, the greater your power will be to change your addiction dance.

This chapter is a transition between an assessment of the factors and conditions that keep you shackled and the steps you can begin to take to heal.

All change begins with hope. If you enter into the recovery process with hope, your journey will be possible. On the other hand, if you enter the recovery process fearful, you may not recover and your journey will be far more difficult.

Chances are you are not feeling very good about yourself. Most men who finally realize they need to address unwanted sexual behavior ask themselves several questions:

- Do I really have a problem?

- Is there something wrong with me?

- Am I the only man doing this?

- Am I a bad person?

The Devil first tries to convince you that your sexual behavior is not bad. "Everyone does it." "It is normal." At the other extreme, the Devil works to convince you that you are worthless and evil. If you simply accept that, "I am an evil person," you may give up hope. Without hope you live in a dark, scary, sad world. With hope, although it may be only a flicker of light far off in the distance, at least there is something to move toward.

Salvation History

Would you be hopeful if you identified with people in salvation history who, like you, had to face a healing process? Yes, salvation history includes a number of key characters who became powerful through the process of personal healing.

King David

King David, the author of the Psalms, is clearly a mainline character in salvation history. Matthew names him in the Lord's ancestral linage. Scripture tells us that the Lord's favor was bestowed upon David many times. Yet, King David was very sexually active, committed serious sexual transgressions, and even murder.

> After he left Hebron, David took more concubines and wives in Jerusalem, and more sons and daughters were born to him. These are the names of the children born to him there: Shammua, Shobab, Nathan, Solomon, Ibhar, Elishua, Nepheg, Japhia, Elishama, Eliada and Eliphelet. (2 Samuel 5:13-16)

> In the spring, at the time when kings go off to war, David sent Joab out with the king's men and the whole Israelite army. They destroyed the Ammonites and besieged Rabbah. But David remained in Jerusalem.

> One evening David got up from his bed and walked around on the roof of the palace. From the roof he saw a woman bathing. The woman was very beautiful, and David sent someone to find out about her. The man said, "Isn't this Bathsheba, the daughter of Eliam and the wife of Uriah the Hittite?" Then David sent messengers to get her. She came to him, and he slept with her. (She had purified herself from her uncleanness.) Then she went back home. The woman conceived and sent word to David, saying, "I am pregnant."

> So David sent this word to Joab: "Send me Uriah the Hittite." And Joab sent him to David. When Uriah came to him, David asked him how Joab was, how the soldiers were and how the war was going. Then David said to Uriah, "Go down to your house and wash your feet." So Uriah left the palace, and a gift from the king was sent after him. But Uriah slept at the entrance to the palace with all his master's servants and did not go down to his house.

> When David was told, "Uriah did not go home," he asked him, "Haven't you just come from a distance? Why didn't you go home?"

> Uriah said to David, "The ark and Israel and Judah are staying in tents, and my master Joab and my lord's men are camped in the open fields. How could I go to my house to eat and drink and lie with my wife? As surely as you live, I will not do such a thing!"

> Then David said to him, "Stay here one more day, and tomorrow I will send you back." So Uriah remained in Jerusalem that day and the next. At David's invitation, he ate and drank with him, and David made him drunk. But in the evening Uriah went out to sleep on his mat among his master's servants; he did not go home.

In the morning David wrote a letter to Joab and sent it with Uriah. In it he wrote, "Put Uriah in the front line where the fighting is fiercest. Then withdraw from him so he will be struck down and die."

So while Joab had the city under siege, he put Uriah at a place where he knew the strongest defenders were. When the men of the city came out and fought against Joab, some of the men in David's army fell; moreover, Uriah the Hittite died. (2 Samuel 11:1-17)

When Uriah's wife heard that her husband was dead, she mourned for him. After the time of mourning was over, David had her brought to his house, and she became his wife and bore him a son. But the thing David had done displeased the LORD. (2 Samuel 11:26)

What are your thoughts as you read the account of David's transgressions?

_____

_____

_____

Do you identify with David? How?

_____

_____

_____

Do you wonder how the Lord could forgive a man like David? Do you wonder how the Lord could forgive you?

_____

_____

_____

Not only was David forgiven, salvation history continues through the heirs of David and Bathsheba.

If God could bless and forgive David of his transgressions, will he forgive you and give you insight in order to recover? How does David's story give you hope?

_____

_____

_____

Apostle Peter

At the time of Christ's greatest need, Peter denied him several times. If there was ever a man who should have given up hope it was Peter; but he didn't. He remained available for forgiveness.

If the God could bless and forgive Peter of his transgressions, will he forgive you and give you the grace to heal? How does Peter's story give you hope?

_____

_____

_____

Apostle Paul

Paul participated in the act of conspiracy to commit murder. He stood by and tended the cloaks of the men who stoned Stephen. He persecuted Christ's followers and yet Christ chose to anoint Paul as His ambassador to bring the Word to the Gentiles.

What are your thoughts about Paul's participation in the murder of Stephen and the persecution of Christ's followers?

_____

_____

_____

Do you identify with Paul? How?

_____

_____

_____

If the Lord could bless a struggling man like Paul to take the "Word" to the Gentiles, what do you think God has in mind for you? Will He forgive you and give you insight to pursue your recovery? How does Paul's story give you hope?

_____

_____

_____

Despite Paul's struggle, he did God's work. If God blessed Paul's struggle, will God also bless your struggle?

_____

_____

_____

Paul found healing and peace. You too can find healing and peace. You too can have hope. You too can change your behavior.

Change the Dance

The change process begins with understanding that the sexual behavior in which you engage is not getting you the satisfaction and the joy of life you desire. Is your sexual behavior causing you more pain than the anticipated pleasure?

_____

_____

_____

The Lord told Paul, "My grace is sufficient for you, for my power is made perfect in weakness." You, too, will need to rely on God to help you change the dance, to make a major change in your life. Although sexual sobriety may be an outcome of therapy, absolute recovery is an illusion. Sexual sobriety without changing the addict's dance does not constitute recovery; it constitutes avoidance. You cannot put a plastic bandage strip on sexual addiction. Plastic bandage strips do not heal the wound. Healing means changing how you think and behave and finding joy in your life.

The remainder of this workbook is intended to help you identify how you plan to change your dance.

Your Summary

What key points did you learn about yourself from this chapter?

Key Point 1:

_____

_____

_____

Key Point 2:

_____

_____

_____

Key Point 3:

_____

_____

_____

Key Point 4:

_____

_____

_____

Key Point 5:

_____

_____

_____

Chapter Eight

Change the Dance

If you were told to just stop sexually acting out, what would be your reply? For some, the answer would be, "I don't know how." Another might say, "I have tried many times and have not succeeded." And another, "I haven't found the answer yet."

In Chapter 8 of the book, *Recovery from Sexual Addiction: A Man's Guide*, you will find helpful information to begin to answer that question. Please read Chapter 8 before doing the exercises in Chapter 8 of this workbook.

Awareness and a Change of Attitude

The process of recovery from sexual addiction is conditioned upon gaining a new sense of awareness and a change of attitude. You become empowered to change the dance when you become more aware of how you became sexually addicted, the factors that keep you sexually addicted, and your role in maintaining your condition. Becoming empowered helps you change your attitude from frustration and despair to one of hope.

The first four chapters of this workbook were designed to help you become aware of what sexual addiction means to you. Below is a summary review of the elements of sexual addiction and how they apply to you.

Summary Review

Affect on my life

I am addicted to . . . (pornography, sexual thinking and fantasy, masturbation, phone sex, massage parlors, escorts)

_____

_____

My sexual addiction has caused problems in my life by . . . (damaging my relationships, my job, and my spirituality; I have contracted VD; I have wasted money)

_____

_____

I have hurt myself by . . . (I am isolated, waste time, and procrastinate; I lead a double life; secrecy keeps me unreal; I lie and believe my own lies)

_____

_____

_____

After acting out, I experience feelings of guilt and shame which lead me to judge myself as . . . (bad, unworthy, disgusting, sinful, sick)

_____

_____

I have tried to stop acting out sexually and the results have been . . . (my addiction has become compulsive and unmanageable; acting out is my greatest need in life; I stop for a while but go back; I have quit trying to stop)

_____

_____

The origin of my addiction

My first memory of being exposed to explicit sexual material or behavior occurred at the age of:

_____

_____

I was exposed to explicit sexual material or behavior by person(s) or circumstances . . .

_____

_____

_____

Feelings I experienced during the event and following the event were . . . (confusion, arousal, excitement, pleasure, guilt, shame)

_____

_____

I did not tell anybody about what happened because . . .

_____

_____

I would have talked to my father about what happened but our relationship was . . .

_____

_____

I remember sex being discussed in our home . . . (never, given a book to read, made to feel dirty)

_____

_____

I began to recreate the feelings I first experienced when I was exposed to age-inappropriate sexual material or behavior by doing . . .

_____

_____

As a teenager I continued to engage in . . . (Alternative: As a teenager I began to engage in . . .)

_____

_____

As an adult I continue to engage in . . .

_____

_____

It would be reasonable to conclude that, "I did not choose to become a sexually-addicted person, but as an adult I can choose to undo what was done to me."

_____

_____

Factors that keep me addicted

"I find it difficult to just stop because my brain has become conditioned to demand satisfaction. My brain tells me I need the chemical flow, the rush caused by sexual stimulation." I feel this is true because . . .

_____

_____

"I frequently engage in sexual thinking or fantasy." I relate to this because . . .

_____

_____

"I don't see the face of a woman. I see her sexual body parts." This describes me because . . .

_____

_____

"Acting out for me is associated with other people, objects (clothing, sex toys, Internet), moods, smells, taste." My environmental sexual triggers are . . .

_____

_____

_____

_____

"I engage in sexual rituals as part of my acting-out cycle. My favorite ritual is . . .

_____

_____

_____

_____

_____

"Each time I act out, I go through an acting-out cycle." My acting-out cycle is . . .

_____

_____

_____

_____

_____

Role of anger

Anger in my life is . . . (often expressed poorly; a real problem; constantly under the surface; a negativity in my life)

_____

_____

Anger contributes to my sexual addiction by . . . (keeping me focused on what is going wrong rather than what is going right, contributing to my depressed mood; being another reason to self medicate)

_____

_____

_____

_____

Role of anxiety

Anxiety in my life is . . . (a real problem; constantly under the surface; negativity in my life)

_____

_____

Anxiety contributes to my sexual addiction by . . . (being a catalyst for me to act out; making masturbation a way to relieve my anxiety; being another reason to self medicate)

_____

_____

Role of low-grade depression

A common characteristic of a sexually-addicted man is to experience low-grade depression most of the time. I identify with this characteristic because . . . (I live most of the time at twenty-point benchmark level, life does not give me the joy I seek; I often feel badly about myself; I have no close friends)

_____

_____

_____

Low-grade depression contributes to my sexual addiction by . . . (being a catalyst for me to act out; using masturbation to relieve my depressed mood; believing that I might as well act out, because nothing else in my life is going well)

_____

_____

_____

_____

_____

Role of isolation

A common characteristic of a sexually-addicted man is to experience isolation, first within his family of origin and later in his adult life. I identify with this characteristic because . . . (I did not have a close relationship with my father; I feel safer when I am alone but I feel lonely; I have few friends; I have no very close friends, etc.)

_____

_____

_____

_____

The most damaging message I took from childhood was . . .

_____

_____

_____

_____

_____

As a child I saw myself as . . . (different; not a part of the in-crowd; ashamed of my sexual behavior; preoccupied with sex)

_____

_____

Isolation contributes to my sexual addiction by . . .

_____

_____

Exceptions

While most sexually-addicted men will identify with most or all of the above profile, I don't identify with . . .

_____

_____

_____

Changing the Dance: New Steps

The previous chapter told us that there is hope. Sexually-addicted men are not bad. They are dealing with a bad problem. God forgave men in salvation history who had greater problems that we have. Now we can explore how we can change the addiction dance.

Following awareness, the most important new step for the addicted man is to learn the difference between white-knuckling and a high-level commitment. White-knuckling is the torture each man puts himself through before acting out. The addicted man tells himself he does not want to act out, but he fails to put the sexual temptation completely out of his mind. He uses interventions that amount to using plastic bandage strips for a serious wound. Plastic bandage strips do nothing but temporarily cover up the wound.

The process of employing temporary interventions is called white-knuckling. Temporary interventions may work from time to time, but long-term sexual sobriety is rarely achieved. The alternative to temporary interventions is making a high-level commitment to end acting out. A high-level commitment consists of making an <u>irrevocable</u> decision to end illicit sexual thinking, fantasy, and behavior.

It is often difficult for the sexually-addicted man to understand the difference between not wanting to act out and making an <u>irrevocable</u> decision to end his addictive behavior. He often convinces himself that not wanting to act out is a high-level commitment. He is then surprised when he falls to temptation. Paradoxically, a man knows he made an irrevocable decision to end his addictive behavior only after experiencing temptation. Once a man makes a high-level commitment, it is significantly easier for him to reject temptation because he has eliminated the possibility of acting out.

A high-level commitment begins with a total rejection of sexual thinking and fantasy. Remember, the mind is the most powerful sex organ a man has. Thus, the battle for sexual sobriety begins in his mind. The highly committed man understands that entertaining sexually stimulating thoughts is simply not acceptable any longer. He learns to recognize (functional awareness) an aberrant thought within a second or two and makes the choice to change his thinking or terminate his fantasy.

A second paradox is this: interventions used by a man who tries to white-knuckle himself to sexual sobriety become useful aids to the highly committed man. For example, a highly committed man will use mental aids to help deal with an environmental temptation. His mantra might be, "I don't want to go there," or, "I am irrevocably committed," or "God made this beautiful woman, she is somebody's daughter." They are no longer plastic bandage strips but expressions of commitment. Other helpful aids to commitment are listed in Appendix A.

While the high-level commitment to end addictive behavior is essential, it is not the only new step a sexually active man needs to take. In the next chapter, other steps will be addressed.

Where are you? Are you white-knuckling or have you made a high-level commitment?

_____

_____

_____

Described the white-knuckling interventions you use. (See Appendix A.)

_____

_____

_____

What stash do you keep hidden away?

_____

_____

_____

What would a high-level commitment look like to you?

_____

_____

_____

How would you change if you made a high-level commitment?

_____

_____

_____

What would your awareness alarm look like if you are highly committed?

_____

_____

_____

Recognize That Addiction Causes More Pain than Pleasure

Attitude change is also essential to make a high-level commitment. The sexually-addicted man sees sex as his most important need. The fact that his compulsive sexual thinking, fantasy, and behavior cause problems in his life, his relationships, and his spirituality are discounted in favor of orgasm. The reality is that orgasms last only a short time. The aftermath of his orgasm plagues a man for a much longer period of time than did his short period of enjoyment. He is beset with feelings of guilt and shame. He feels bad about his inability to control his thinking and behavior. He realizes, on some level, his life is in disarray.

Note: Orgasm as part of a loving marital relationship does not have shame and guilt consequences.

As a man approaches a high-level commitment he begins to understand his search for sexual pleasure causes more pain than it is worth. He realizes his pain/pleasure equation is out of balance. He finally comprehends the amount of pain he experiences is no longer reasonable. It is a turning point for the sexually-addicted man to come to the understanding that there is more pain than pleasure in his addiction. It is also an important change in attitude toward his behavior.

How about you? What pain is your sexual addiction causing you?

_____

_____

_____

How would your life be different if you were not experiencing this pain?

_____

_____

_____

Is it time for you to give up this pain?

_____

_____

_____

Address Environmental Temptation

Visual sexual stimulation is a curse to the sexually-addicted man. Even when a man plans to seek sexual sobriety, the media, television, newspaper, and billboard advertising all sell sex. For the sexually-addicted man, the Internet, pornographic movies, and TV fuel his lust. The sexually-addicted man must change his environment to reduce sexual stimulation.

What environmental conditions facilitate your addiction?

_____

_____

_____

_____

If you made a high-level commitment what changes would you make in your environment?

_____

_____

_____

_____

Your Summary

What key points did you learn about yourself from this chapter?

Key Point 1:

_____

_____

_____

Key Point 2:

_____

_____

_____

Key Point 3:

_____

_____

_____

Key Point 4:

_____

_____

_____

Key Point 5:

_____

_____

_____

Chapter Nine

Healthy Lifestyle

The previous chapter explored essential elements related to recovery from sexual addiction.

- The first of these is to make a high-level commitment to end acting out.

- The second is to change your attitude, that is, understand that your addiction is causing you more pain than pleasure.

- The third is to change your environment when it facilitates acting out.

This chapter calls you to support your high-level commitment by living a healthy lifestyle. Since the sexually-addicted man typically lives in isolation and low-grade depression, key to long-term recovery is changing one's lifestyle to forgo isolation and low-grade depression. The addicted man must also address codependency in his marriage as well as his relationship with his God. The last element is to employ a support network to guard against a relapse.

A healthier lifestyle helps to reduce anger, anxiety, and depression, and ultimately will reduce acting out. If you reduce negativity in your life and thus the need to medicate your pain, your entire life will become more satisfying. Addressing sexual addiction is not one dimensional. Addressing sexual addiction means choosing to become a healthier person physically and mentally.

In Chapter 9 of the book, *Recovery from Sexual Addiction: A Man's Guide*, you will find helpful information to help you live a healthier lifestyle. Read Chapter 9 before doing the exercises in Chapter 9 of this workbook.

Coming Out of Isolation

"I tend to live in isolation. I live in my head. Sexual fantasy and thinking dominate my brain waves. Unfortunately, I have valued my addiction more than my relationships." Do these statements apply to you? If yes, how? If not, why?

_____

_____

_____

"I live in two worlds. In one world, I want other people to see me as a good guy, a contributing member to society. In my other world, I am a shame-based person who is fearful of others seeing the real me and learning my secrets." Do these statements apply to you? If yes, how? If not, why?

_____

_____

_____

"I have few or no close friends. I don't let my male friends know about my sexual thinking, fantasies, and behavior." Do these statements apply to you? If yes, how? If not, why?

_____

_____

_____

Is it time to come out of your isolation and to live a joyful life? The following are some changes for your consideration.

Coming out of isolation by cultivating a strong male friendship

It is so important to cultivate a strong male friendship—a friendship which, in time, will allow you to share the real you, your problems, and your journey. Life is often a paradox. It is precisely the need to share one's weakness, the need to allow another male to pierce the veil of the addicted man's secret world, that makes the effort to find and make a new male friend so valuable. It is by sharing and thus defusing one's shame that begins to reduce the underlying need to medicate one's pain by engaging in sexual behavior.

"I fear sharing my weakness, my addiction, with another man. I fear rejection and even more isolation." Do these statements apply to you? If yes, describe your fear. If not, why?

_____

_____

_____

If the above statement applies to you, let's test reality. Do you really think it is a sign of weakness to be vulnerable to another man? Time and time again men have reported that when they are vulnerable to another man they find even more respect, and often the other man becomes vulnerable too. Perhaps you can be a blessing to the man with whom you share.

Are you willing to come out of isolation by cultivating a strong male relationship?

_____

_____

_____

How would you cultivate a strong male friendship? What steps would you take?

_____

_____

_____

Coming out of isolation by improving family relationships

Relationships sexually-addicted men have with family members often range from nonexistent to shallow. Since childhood relationships were weak, it follows that adult relationships are also weak. Furthermore, the sexually-addicted man fears exposing his shameful secrets to those he believes are more judgmental than even his friends.

Again, it is precisely the need to pierce the shame barrier that begins to defuse the underlying need to medicate pain. If the sexually-addicted man fears intimacy with family members, it is likely that family members fear intimacy with him. Family healing is an opportunity to create new possibilities for joy.

"I am fearful of sharing myself with my family members. I fear rejection and even more isolation." Do these statements apply to you? If yes, how? If not, why?

_____

_____

_____

Again, let's test reality: Do you really think all members of your family will reject you? Even if they did, how much worse off would you be than you are today?

_____

_____

_____

What rewards do you perceive are possible from gaining a deeper level of intimacy with your family members?

_____

_____

_____

Are you willing to come out of isolation by cultivating a new friendship with one or more family members?

_____

_____

_____

How would you cultivate a new friendship with one or more family members? Which family member would you approach first? What steps would you take?

_____

_____

_____

Note: Sharing information with family members related to your sexual addiction is a secondary objective. The primary objective is to come out of isolation by fostering healthy family relationships. While, in many case, it is desirable for family members to know who you are and your weaknesses, sharing your sexual addiction is not mandatory. That knowledge is shared when you feel it will contribute to a deeper understanding and intimacy.

Coming out of isolation by improving relationships with spouse and children

"When I think about it, my relationship with my wife is based on sex. When we engage in sexual activity, I am satisfied with our relationship." Do these statements of apply to you? If yes, how? If not, why?

_____

_____

_____

"I fear sharing my secrets with my wife because I know she will try to fix me. I know I am bad, but I hate it when she points it out to me. I fear her rejection." Do these statements apply to you? If yes, how? If not, why?

_____

_____

_____

Again, let's test reality: Do you really think your wife will reject you? Even if she did, how much worse off would you be than you are today?

_____

_____

_____

"I wish my wife was my best friend, but I really don't know what a best friend is. While we live in the same house, I often feel we are distant relatives living under the same roof." Do these statements apply to you? If yes, how? If not, why?

_____

_____

_____

What rewards do you perceive are possible from gaining a deeper level of intimacy with your wife and children?

_____

_____

_____

_____

Are you willing to come out of isolation by cultivating a new friendship with your wife and children?

_____

_____

_____

_____

How would you cultivate a new friendship with your wife and children? What steps would you take?

_____

_____

_____

_____

Improving family relationships with your spouse and children is a major step in coming out of isolation. Perhaps it is the most important. Sharing the knowledge of your sexual addiction with your wife for the first time is best done with the help of a competent therapist who understands sexual addiction. The therapist can help normalize the disclosure and explain the nature of sexual addiction to your spouse. In addition, the book, *Getting the Love You Want,* by Harville Hendrix, is helpful to many men.

Giving-up Depressed Mood

How would you characterize your depressed mood? List below the conditions you experience as symptoms of depressed mood. For example, do you focus on what is going wrong rather than on what is going right? Are you unable to sleep and eat healthily regularly? Do you tolerate your day rather than experience the joy of being alive? Are you often sad? Do you frequently waste time or procrastinate? Do you seek sex to medicate depressed mood?

Condition 1

_____

_____

Condition 2

_____

_____

Condition 3

_____

_____

Condition 4

_____

_____

Condition 5

_____

_____

It might seem strange to ask you the question, "Do you like to live in your depressed mood?" Most men would be quick to say, "Of course not." But the reality is, many men actually choose to live in their depressed mood rather than take steps to change. One man said, "I moved into my rut, and I furnished the walls." He knew what his rut looked like, for he had lived in his rut for many years. While the sexually-addicted man knows the color of his rut's walls, he is fearful of the unknown outside of his rut. It takes great courage and discipline to move out of one's rut. It takes giving up a comfortable place for one that is less comfortable, at least initially.

Do you have the courage and discipline to move out of your rut? What would you have to give up?

_____

_____

Choose to take steps to live at a forty-point benchmark level

From a practical point of view, the sexually-addicted man needs to choose a healthier lifestyle simply to make the high from acting out a lesser enticement. If he begins to live closer to forty, the need to relieve pain of living at twenty is reduced. Living at forty not only relieves depressed mood, but also helps the addicted man to give up his isolation.

While the changes needed to live at forty may be different for each man, below are some examples for your personal consideration.

- Engage in healthy recreation. Carve out a period of each week to enjoy life such as biking, walking, playing with one's children, taking one's spouse out to dinner.

- Become active in a club or church.

- Engage your wife or friend in good conversation. Start with fifteen minutes a day and continue to add time. Aim for an hour of good conversation each day.

- Call one or more friends every day.

- Cultivate strong male and family member friendships.

- Focus on what is going right in your life, not what is going wrong.

- Serve others. As part of coming out of isolation, a man can choose to be of service to others. For example, consider serving periodically at a soup kitchen, coaching a sports team, or joining a prison ministry.

- Consider consulting your doctor about your depressed mood or chronic anxiety. Your doctor may prescribe appropriate medication. Such medication may be a valuable catalyst to stabilize your life so that, in therapy, you can focus on your sexual addiction rather than other stressors.

What activities would help you move out of your rut?

Activity 1

_____

_____

Activity 2

_____

_____

Activity 3

_____

_____

Activity 4

_____

_____

Activity 5

_____

_____

A Close Relationship with God

Rarely does a sexually-addicted man have a close relationship with God. He fears a God of punishment because of his addiction. It's difficult for the addicted man to view his God as loving when he himself doesn't really understand what it is to have been loved unconditionally by his family of origin. He also does not know how to be loving in his human relationships. His childhood learning model was deficient.

What is your relationship with God? What are the characteristics of God in your life? Be honest.

For example, is God distant like your father was distant to you? Is God vengeful? Is God's love for you conditional on how well you behave sexually? Do you find it difficult to understand how God could love you unconditionally, even when you act out? Is God someone whom you want as a friend, but not now?

1. God for me is . . .

_____

_____

2. God for me is . . .

_____

_____

3. God for me is . . .

_____

_____

4. God for me is . . .

_____

_____

5. God for me is . . .

_____

_____

Change your relationship with God

A sexually-addicted man's relationship with God is incomplete. He feels God's love for him is conditional on his sexual sobriety. How can a man have hope when he does not feel the love that God has for him?

Perhaps the most important change a sexually-addicted man needs to make is to change his thinking about his relationship with God. When the sexually-addicted man sees God as his greatest cheerleader in the battle with addiction, there is a refuge for his struggle and pain. Ultimately, as taught in Twelve Step programs, the addicted man understands he is powerless over his addiction. He learns the power of surrender. He places himself in the hands of his God. While God will not do the man's work, God will provide insight sufficient for him to do his recovery work.

What would a loving God look like to you?

_____

_____

_____

How can you change your thinking to understand God is your greatest cheerleader? Can you believe God is sad when you fall, but never ceases to love you?

_____

_____

_____

Describe God as you want Him to join you on your journey.

_____

_____

_____

Develop a Support Network

The sexually-addicted man cannot go alone. He needs a support network. Below are some possibilities.

- Twelve Step Programs

- Accountability Partner

- Individual Counseling

- Group Counseling

- Family Counseling

- Marriage Therapy

- Targeted reading programs

- Celebrate Recovery

- One Man's Battle Program

- Targeted Bible Study

I am considering the following as my support network:

Support Network 1

_____

_____

Support Network 2

_____

_____

Support Network 3

_____

_____

Support Network 4

_____

_____

Your Summary

What key points did you learn about yourself from this chapter?

Key Point 1:

_____

_____

_____

Key Point 2:

_____

_____

_____

Key Point 3:

_____

_____

_____

Key Point 4:

_____

_____

_____

Key Point 5:

_____

_____

_____

Appendix A

Interventions and Aids to Commitment

Over the years, men in counseling have found effective interventions or aids to commitment. Since every man is unique, you will need to find which of those offered below help you. Don't be surprised to find you need unique interventions or aids to commitment. Interventions are analogous to plastic bandage strips. They are temporary coverings. They do not cure the wound. The use of interventions alone does not constitute a recovery program. On the other hand once a high-level commitment is made, aids to commitment support the fundamental decision to renounce acting out.

Paradoxically, once a high-level commitment is made, these same interventions become valuable aids in support of your decision to permanently change your sexual thinking and behavior. As aids they are part of your recovery program.

- Actively participate in Twelve Step and counseling programs.

- Be accountable to yourself—make a conscious choice to eliminate sexual thinking, fantasy, or thoughts.

- Disclose your addiction to an accountability partner or a good male friend. With the aid of a therapist disclose your addiction behavior to your spouse.

- Develop a support network to call in the time of sexual urges. Reach out—call a good male friend or an accountability partner in time of deteriorating mood or when sexual urges begin your acting-out ritual.

- Be aware of your own needs, resentments, stresses, anxiety, and loneliness and how each feeling sets the stage for acting-out sexually. Deal with underlying issues through counseling.

- Take care of your HALTs (Hunger, Anger, Loneliness, and Tiredness). When the addict is in one of the HALT states, his propensity to engage in unwanted sexual behavior greatly escalates. Become aware of the symptoms of the approaching HALT state and have a counter measure preplanned to avert it.

- Medicate anxiety. If you feel high-level anxiety and to experience relief you masturbate, anti-anxiety medication may help until the source of anxiety is removed. High levels of chronic anxiety is toxic both to mental and physical health. (Some medications are addictive and should be taken only under medical supervision. Consult a psychiatrist for a full evaluation and an appropriate prescription.)

- Become aware of your various acting-out rituals and learn to recognize when a ritual is beginning. After you experience an acting-out incidence and while the memory is fresh, write down the various steps which led you to act out. Focus on early steps and identify a step at which you became aware you were heading toward a relapse. Preplan an intervention for that stage.

- Become fully aware of the persons, places, feelings, thinking, or things that lead you to act out. Preplan interventions that will diffuse each of these conditions.

- If you are more likely to act out when you are alone, plan ahead not to be alone.

- Become aware of your triggers. Reject them before they happen.

- Put a mantra on your computer, for example, "I will not use this computer to gain access to pornographic material."

- Put a pornography filter on your computer.

- Do not watch TV programs with sexual content. Alternatively, record TV programs you like to watch and fast-forward through sexually disturbing material, ads, or other difficult parts.

- Think through the mantra, "Where am I heading?", when you feel the urge to begin your acting-out ritual. Form a mantra that works for you, for example, "I don't have the right to go there!" or "Don't go there," or "I don't have to be a pursuer of my past."

- Just say no! Make a high level commitment to say no.

- Verbalize cognitive thinking to defuse sexual feelings. In other words, talk out loud to yourself.

- Use an alternative healthy fantasy in place of a sexual fantasy. For example, play fantasy football in your head, play a round of golf in your head, or remember a time when you felt relaxed and enjoyed life.

- Plan more healthy personal time to deal with stress. For example, regular exercise reduces stress. In time of a sexual urge use an immediate exercise intervention such as twenty pushups.

- Intimacy does not equal sex. Learn to practice and enjoy non-sexual intimacy with your spouse. For example, take a walk together, talk about what is important to each

Paul Becker, LPC

of you, and plan other activities that build your relationship. Work to make your spouse your best friend.

- Spend quality time with your family.

- Understand the factors that foster your choice to live at the forty benchmark and program them into your life.

- Treat yourself to small rewards for not acting out for a set period of time, let's say, a week. One man's self-reward is one hour of shooting pool for every four days of sobriety.

- Understand the degree of pleasure derived from acting out in comparison to the pain of guilt, shame, and time wasted. If the balance is negative, ask yourself why you want to do something that is causing more pain than gain.

- Dispute illogical thinking. If you are lying to yourself or engaging in illogical thinking, admit it and look for truth.

- Learn to bounce your eyes away from sexually titillating images or persons.

- Understand that sexual temptation will continue throughout your life and learn to turn away.

- If you are married, focus on transferring your thinking and your gaze to your wife.

- Instead of seeing a woman as a sex object, see her as someone's mother or daughter. Thank God for making a beautiful woman and let it go.

- Attach a person to a woman or sexual image. See the humanness of the person by focusing on the person's face, eyes, smile, and facial expressions.

- Use a journal to keep in touch with reality—to track moods, lies, triggers, or rituals.

- Work to gain greater awareness of yourself and the world.

- Carry a picture of your family. Take it out when your feel the urge to act out.

- Make physical adjustments to preclude your acting-out ritual—get rid of cable TV or the Internet or choose safe routes.

- Trash stash. *Stash* is sexually stimulating material hidden away in anticipation of a future time of need. Examples include a hidden porno magazine or an Internet URL to connect to sexually stimulating web pages tucked away on your PC.

- Address other addictions—alcohol, drugs, gambling, eating disorders, anger, etc.

- 134 -

- Imagine God's presence in the room when you feel the urge to act out.

- Take a ten minute walk. That is, remove yourself physically from the locus of your sexual urge.

- Make prayer or other spiritual reading part of your life. Carry a motivational verse or scriptural passage to bring you back to reality when you are feeling the urge to act out.

- Play spiritual music to ward off the urge to act out when you are alone.

- Surrender—In the Twelve Step traditions understand and acknowledge it will take both you and God to travel your recovery journey. Ask God's help—understand that the self is powerless.

- Dedicate your home to your God and refrain from acting out there.

- Plan and practice an active spiritual life.

- Have spiritual reading handy in times of sexual urges.

- Learn to forgive yourself.

- If you find yourself living below the forty benchmark for weeks at a time, consider going on depression medication combined with individual therapy.

- If you find yourself engaging in outbursts of anger, consider individual therapy.

- If you find your unwanted sexual behavior is continuing, consider individual therapy.

- Make a list from above of interventions you want to use, post the list where you normally act out, and use it to help yourself.

Note: Each item in the list above either addresses quality of life or actions one can take at the time of an urge to act out. The road to recovery must address both. In the short run, one needs interventions to help to reject a specific temptation. When making your list of interventions, make two. Include on one list those interventions that address your quality of life. On the other list include interventions which address specific sexual urges. Both lists should be readily available. In time of need, it is difficult to think through alternative interventions. A preplanned list facilitates the use of an appropriate intervention as opposed to acting out.

Which interventions did you choose?

Intervention 1

_____

_____

Intervention 2

_____

_____

Intervention 3

_____

_____

Intervention 4

_____

_____

Intervention 5

_____

_____

Intervention 6

_____

_____

Intervention 7

_____

_____